Study Guide to Accompany

WHITNEY   HAMILTON

Understanding Nutrition

THIRD EDITION

PREPARED BY

Lorraine E. Bailey, B.S., M.S.
Cuesta College

WEST PUBLISHING COMPANY
St. Paul · New York · Los Angeles · San Francisco

Contents

Preface

To **The** Student

It is stated that a person with average retention skills hears
an idea once and within 24 hours 25% is forgotten, in 48 hours
50% is forgotten, if four days 85% is forgotten and in sixteen
days 98% is forgotten. Ever wonder why "cramming" never works?
BUT, if you hear something six times, with sleep intervals in
between, 63% will be <u>retained</u> <u>indefinitely</u>!

Because we hope your study of nutrition will be an experience
that will help you--and your family--be healthier and more
productive the rest of your life, we don't want this to be just
another course you pass to "get a grade." We have, therefore,
designed a method to make it easier to study, understand, retain,
apply <u>and</u> get a better grade in your nutrition course. This
study guide is planned to involve as many of your senses as
possible so you can use your study time to better advantage and
it also will provide excellent review of important material
before a quiz or an examination.

You are fortunate to have your text, <u>Understanding Nutrition</u>,
to lead you to an in-depth acquaintanceship with the science of
nutrition. Complex ideas have been treated simply and clearly;
you can easily understand them if you provide the necessary
attention.

The material in the study guide parallels the material found in
the textbook. By using both of these books, you will find
mastery and retention of the necessary information much easier.

To help you apply what you have learned, some practical recipes
have been provided. It is hoped you will be motivated to
improve your own eating habits parallel to your new knowledge
about the importance of food to the maintenance and repair of
your body. "You are what you eat," "**food** becomes you." The
first step in effective living is to value yourself and realize
the importance of caring for your body. If it falls apart,
what are you going to live in the rest of your life?

It has been said that the human body is the only incredible
"machine," but it is one that lacks an owner's manual. Your
nutrition course helps make up for the lack.

Best wishes for success in this pursuit of learning more about
yourself.

L. E. B.

To Use This Study Guide:

1) Read the objectives (You Will Learn. . .) presented on the first page of each chapter of the study guide.

2) Read the entire chapter or chapter summary.

3) Fill in the blanks of the Study Guide Questions from the text.

4) Check your filled-in blanks with the Study Guide Answers and correct questions missed or fill in missing information.

5) Reread the chapter summary and immediately take the Self-Test.

6) Check your answers in the Self-Test Answers section and re-study questions you were unsure of or missed.

You should be able to remember information and be well prepared for testing by applying this study process.

Reading the entire chapter first is highly recommended. Rather than trying to memorize, read it as rapidly as possible for general understanding. Then go through it again, filling in answers in the study guide to help summarize important points.

The study guide questions can serve as a practical review for examinations. Add to your review the lecture material your instructor has stressed.

Welcome to the fascinating world of nutrition; theory and application!

Acknowledgements

It is wonderful to find a textbook that provides information that can be immediately applied to daily living yet clearly contribute to scientific understanding. Your textbook's authors have provided this remarkable combination.

Developing written material is difficult at best, especially when undertaken in addition to a full teaching load. However, I am pleased to be able to offer some practical applications of nutrition which students ask for. Also, in my own nutrition consulting practice I find that "you are what you eat" needs interpreting into the preparation of food in a practical and enjoyable way that can fit into busy schedules and limited budgets.

In acknowledging the people who have been most influential and supportive of my special interest in foods and nutrition I have to start with my sons, Bruce and Ronald Hensel whom I loved enough to learn to prepare healthful food even when it would have been easier to serve the "junk" that was popular. Having a healthy family has been my finest achievement and I would like to help others discover this blessing.

Special thanks to my parents, Edith and Harold Wicht, for setting a good example, and especially to my mother for teaching me the real joy of nutrition--caring for oneself and others.

There is no way I could thank my friend Carol Bower enough for putting this manuscript on the computer and giving the project priority time in her busy schedule as homemaker and student.

I am very grateful to my husband, Gordon Bailey, for his patient support and to all others who have helped make possible this opportunity to help others in understanding and applying nutrition.

Lorraine E. Bailey, B.S., M.S.
Home Economist
Cuesta College

CHAPTER 1

Introduction to Nutrition

YOU WILL LEARN...

1. That you are made entirely of what you have eaten.

2. That a nutrient is a substance obtained from food and used in the body to promote growth, maintenance or repair.

3. The six classes of nutrients and that all foods contain a combination of these.

4. The chemist's definition of the word "organic."

5. What nutrients produce energy.

6. The definition of the term <u>calorie,</u> or <u>kcalorie,</u> and how energy in food is measured.

7. The important roles of vitamins, minerals, and water.

8. How food group plans evolved and how to use them to improve your own diet.

9. What the RDA stands for, how it is determined, and what U.S. RDA means.

10. How nutritional guidelines set for healthy people in the U.S. compare with those of Canada and the rest of the world.

11. To differentiate among dietary recommendations, dietary goals and dietary guidelines.

12. How to use the Four Food Group Plan and the Exchange System.

CHAPTER 1:   INTRODUCTION TO NUTRITION

HIGHLIGHT 1A: NATURAL FOODS

13.   The difference between organic, natural and health food.

14.   What consumers need to know about "health foods."

15.   The greatest advantage of organic farming.

Highlight 1B: VITAMIN SUPPLEMENTS

16.   The existence of nutritional individuality.

17.   How vitamins are promoted.

18.   What to watch out for in purchasing supplements.

19.   The risks of mineral – vitamin toxicity.

CHAPTER 1: INTRODUCTION TO NUTRITION

INTRODUCTION TO NUTRITION

1. It has been said that you are what you EAT, food becomes you.

2. You are a collection of MOLECULES that move, arranged into cells, tissues, and ORGANS.

3. The parts are continually being process using NUTRIENT and ENERGY derived from nutrients.

4. Your oldest red blood cell is only 120 days old and the lining of your digestive tract is renewed every 3 days.

5. You are made entirely of what you have EATEN.

6. A simple definition of the science of nutrition is: The study of the NUTRIENT in food and the body's handling of these NUTRIENT.

THE NUTRIENTS

7. A nutrient is a substance obtained from food and used in the body to promote growth, MAINTENANCE, or repair.

8. An "essential nutrient" is one the body cannot make for itself in sufficient quantity, but has to be obtained from FOOD.

9. There are six classes of nutrients, and the study of nutrition revolves around them. They are:
(MEMORIZE FOR EXAM)

CARBOHYDRATES	WATER
FAT	VITAMINS
PROTEIN	MINERAL

3

10. If your body underwent chemical analysis, the largest component found would be _____WATER_____.

11. Besides nutrients, other things found in food and in your body could include intentional _additives_ and incidental _pollutants_.

12. If a food is burned in air the water evaporates, and the organic compounds are oxidized to _gas_, leaving a residue of _ash_.

13. The correct definition of the word <u>organic</u> is simply that it contains _carbon_ atoms.

14. All foods and vitamins are _organic_ even synthetic products, so there is no reason to believe organic means superior.

15. While carbohydrate, fat, protein, and vitamins are organic, _mineral_ and _water_ are not.

16. The energy nutrients are _protein_, _fat_, and _carbohydrates_.

17. Energy nutrients are _oxidized_ during metabolism, providing energy the body can use.

18. Oxidation in the body is a chemical process that releases chemical and _mechanical_ energy rather than light and heat, like the burning of wood.

19. Metabolism is the name given to processes in which _nutrients_ are rearranged into body structures or broken down to use for _energy_.

THE ENERGY NUTRIENTS

20. No energy is produced from _vitamin_ or _mineral_ because they do not oxidize in the human body.

21. The amount of energy released from food is measured in calories which should be written _kcalories_.

22. A calorie is the amount of heat necessary to raise the temperature of a _gram_ of water _one_ degree Centigrade. Because the calorie is such a small unit, food energy is measured in thousands of calories, or kcalories

CHAPTER 1: INTRODUCTION TO NUTRITION

23. When the United States goes metric, we may be using _kilojoules_ as units of energy.

24. Alcohol also yields _energy_, but does not promote growth, maintenance, or repair of body tissues.

25. Practically all foods contain mixtures of all three _energy_ nutrients, but many are identified by the one present in the largest amount.

26. Two exceptions to this rule are sugar, which is almost pure _carbohydrate_, and oil, which is almost pure _fat_.

27. The energy nutrients are very large molecules, maybe containing as many as 7,000 atoms. When they are broken down they yield a lot of _energy_ for our use.

28. An average serving of food or juice is about _100_ grams; one teaspoon of any dry powder such as flour about _5_ grams.

29. If you could purify the energy nutrients in your daily diet, they would fill two or three measuring _cups_.

30. Vitamins are also _organic_ compounds. There are at least _15_ different vitamins, all with special functions in the body.

31. Vitamins have several important properties. They yield no energy when oxidized but because they are organic they are _distructible_.

32. Vitamins can easily be destroyed by excess alkali, air, heat, or _light_.

33. The two classes of vitamins are water-soluble and _fat_ -soluble. This distinction determines how the body absorbs, transports, stores, and excretes them.

THE MINERALS

34. Minerals are _inorganic_ compounds, smaller than vitamins, and are found in simple forms in foods. There are _21_ different minerals important in nutrition.

35. Minerals are _inorganic_, because they have never been a part of a living thing.

36. Minerals, unlike vitamins, are _indiahuctible_ and need not be handled with special care.

37. Minerals associate with water and influence its distribution into different body compartments. Minerals also influence the _acid_ - _base_ balance of the body.

WATER

38. The major part of every body tissue is formed by _Water_. Water is inorganic and yields no energy.

39. You need about _ten_ times as much water as you need energy nutrients.

40. Body water comes from three sources:
     1. Drinking water,
     2. Water contained in foods,
     3. Water generated from the oxidation of _energy_ nutrients.

41. Water is excreted in four ways:
     1. Urination,
     2. Losses in the feces,
     3. Evaporation from the skin,
     4. Evaporation from the _lungs_.

FOOD GROUP PLANS

42. Diet planning principles are:

     1. A _Adequacy_   C _Calorie Control_
         B _Balance_   V _Variety_

43. The Four Food Group Plan specifies:
     1. two servings of _Protein food_
     2. two servings of _calcium reach food_
     3. four servings of _fruit & Vegetable_
     4. four servings of _whole grain, cereab & bread_

44. Miscellaneous items do not fit into the four food group system if they are not foods, if their nutrient content is too low to qualify them for inclusion in a specific group, or if their nutrient content has been greatly diluted by _sugar_, _fat_, or water.

45. The Four Food Group Plan is quite _flexible_ and can be adapted to different national and cultural menus. Most people _do not_ (do/do not) follow it.

46. Even if you do follow it faithfully you can still be short in vitamin B , magnesium, iron, zinc and vitamin _E_.

47. The Modified Four Food Group Plan published in 1978 recommends adding two servings of _legume_, portion size _3/4 cup_, and increasing the two servings of meat, fish, or poultry to _3 oz._ each.

48. In addition, breads and cereals chosen are to be _whole grain_, not enriched, and one serving of fat or oil is to be added for vitamin _, E_.

49. While it is possible to make low-kcalorie choices in the Four Food Group Plan and eat all recommended servings at a kcalorie cost of 1,200, eating everything in the Modified Four Group Plan brings the kcalories up to _2,200_. There is not much leeway for free food choices, but there is a virtual guarantee of diet _adequacy_.

50. Many experiments show that the addition of _legume_ to the daily meal plan makes the needed difference between barely adequate and ample. Tofu, peanut butter, bean sprouts, lentils, peas, and all kinds of beans are members of this group.

51. There are _two_ major classes of vegetarians with many variations. The _lacto-ovo_ vegetarian uses milk and eggs. The _vegan_ is a strict vegetarian and needs to take a vitamin _B_ supplement.

Note: Further study will indicate that the vegetarian may be more at risk lacking vitamin B-12, zinc, and iron than adequate protein.

NUTRIENT DENSITY

52. The concept of _nutrient density_ may become the basis for a new kind of food labeling.

53. Foods that provide more nutrients than kcalories, relative to a person's need, qualify to be labeled _nutritious_ _food_.

54.   An adequate diet is one that provides all of the
_____necessary_____ nutrients and _____kcalories_____ necessary to
maintain health and body weight.

55.   Ideally, a diet will be _____optimal_____, not just adequate, and
support the best possible state of health.

56.   Protective or _____foundation_____ _____foods_____ are nutrient-
_____dense_____ foods around which a nutritious diet can be
constructed. These foods are: milk, cheese, meat, fish,
poultry, eggs, legumes, nuts, fruits, vegetables, and
_____grains_____.

EXCHANGE SYSTEMS

If the exchange lists bother you, think of them as lists of
alternatives or substitutions. All the food portions on one
list have approximately the same number of kcalories and the
same amounts of energy nutrients. HINT: The key to following
the exchange system is in using "the amount of a food specified"
since if you ate twice as much of something listed it would no
longer be equal to the others.

57.   There are _____six_____ lists of foods in the exchange system:
_____milk_____, _____vegetable_____, _____fruit_____, bread,
meat, and fat.

      Please note that serving sizes are different on some of the
      lists from those of the Four Food Group system. Also,
      some of the foods are classified differently.

58.   Cheese is classed as a _____meat_____ in the exchange system
and as a dairy product in the Four Food Group system.

59.   If you know the number of grams of the energy nutrients in
a certain food you can easily calculate the kcalories.
MEMORIZE that:
      1 g carbohydrate is _____4_____ kcal.
      1 g fat is _____9_____ kcal.
      1 g protein is _____4_____ kcal.
Later on you will learn that alcohol is 7 kcal per gram,
which makes alcoholic beverages costly in kcalories.

60.   The user of the exchange system is encouraged to think of
skim milk as _____milk_____ and of whole milk as milk with
added _____fat_____.

61.   Vegetables such as _____corn_____ and _____lima_____ _____beans_____ are
listed with bread because of their carbohydrate content.

62.   Nutritional adequacy can be assured with either the Four Food Group Plan or the Exchange system, but the one more easily used to limit kcalories is the _exchange list_ .

RECOMMENDED NUTRIENT INTAKES

63.   Many countries have developed _dietary_ standards. Three are discussed in the text: those of the United States, of _Canada_ , and of the World Health Organization.

64.   RDA stands for _Recomended_ _Dietary_ _ALLAWONCE_ .

65.   There are three parts to the RDA table. The main one includes recommendations for protein, ten vitamins, and six minerals. Another table specifies energy needs for people of both sexes at different ages, and another presents tentative recommendations for _12_ more vitamins and minerals.

66.   These figures are reviewed and revised about every _5_ years.

67.   The figures are based on AVAILABLE _scientific_ evidence. They are recommendations for healthy persons only and are not minimum _requirement_ .

68.   There are separate recommendations for _different_ sets of people.

The Setting of Recommended Allowances

69.   The RDA cannot be taken literally by any one _individual_ .

70.   The RDA are not for the _restoration_ of health.

The RDA for Energy

71.   The energy RDA is set at _mean_ .

72.   No RDA is set for _carbohydrate_ or _fat_ .

The U.S. RDA

73.   The term U.S. RDA appears on _food_ _labels_ .

74. For most nutrients, the U.S. RDA is the same as the *RDA* for an adult _____man_____.

75. The woman's RDA is used for _____iron_____.

    Note: If a product is intended for babies or children only, its label shows the RDA for that age group.

Other Recommendations

76. The Canadian recommendations are slightly different from ours because the Canadian authorities interpreted the ___data___ differently, and because conditions in Canada are not the same as available in the United States.

77. FAO stands for the Food and *Agriculture* Organization.

78. The WHO is the World ___Health___ Organization.

79. The FAO/WHO recommendations are considered sufficient for "nearly _all_ _people_."

80. They are sometimes _higher_, usually _lower_, than the RDA.

81. FAO/WHO recommends a _higher_ intake of protein because the quality protein people consume world-wide is lower than that of protein in the United States.

82. The United States has a _higher_ calcium recommendation than FAO/WHO to keep the calcium intake in balance with the ___high___ phosphorus and protein intakes of its people.

EVALUATION OF NUTRITION STATUS

83. A primary deficiency is a nutrient deficiency caused by inadequate ___dietry___ ___intake___ of a nutrient.

84. A secondary deficiency is caused by something other than a _nutrient_.

85. In the early stages, before signs are obvious, a deficiency is called a ___subclinical___ deficiency.

86. Taking a diet history is a good way to discover *deficiencies* before the end stage is reached.

87. There can be pitfalls in doing a self study. For example:
    a. You may not be careful in recording amounts eaten
        and doing the correct mathematical calculations.
    b. Values in food tables are not absolute because
        foods can vary.
    c. Values assume reasonable care in food preparation.
    d. You are assumed to be ___healthy___.
    e. No provisions are made for medications that
        interfere with nutrition.
    f. It is assumed you will absorb and use the nutrients
        ___normally___.

88. Another method of evaluation is the physical ___examination___
    in which parts of the body such as hair, eyes, skin,
    posture, tongue, fingernails, are inspected for clues to
    nutrition problems.

89. A third way is to conduct ___laboratory___ tests on blood,
    urine, or body tissues.

90. Anthropometric measures such as height, weight, and other
    measurements can detect ___growth___ failure in children and
    wasting or ___swelling___ in adults.

DIETARY GUIDELINES

91. Diseases arising in part from excesses in kcalories, fat,
    salt, sugar and protein have prompted government groups to
    make dietary ___recomendation___ to their people.

92. In 1976, there were <u>Dietary Recommendations for</u>
    ___canadian___.

93. In 1977, the <u>Dietary Goals for the</u> ___United___
    ___STATE___ were published.

94. In 1980, the <u>Dietary Guidelines for</u> ___American___ were
    published.

95. These sets of guidelines differ somewhat from each other,
    but there is more agreement than ___disagreement___.

96. Review the seven U.S. <u>Dietary Goals.</u> One of them has to do
    with energy, two with carbohydrate, three with fat, and one
    with ___salt___.

97. The most dramatic dietary change recommended was that we
    should increase our consumption of ___complex___
    carbohydrates.

98. The same general principles are stressed in the <u>Goals</u> as in the <u>Guidelines.</u>   The <u>Goals</u> state them in terms of _____nutrient_____, The <u>Guidelines</u> translate them into _____food_____.

99. The U.S. Senate, Select Committee on Nutrition and Human Needs, that recommended the <u>Dietary Goals,</u> has since been _____disbanded_____.

100. The <u>Dietary Guidelines</u> were produced by the USDHHS and the _____USDA_____.

101. The seventh Guideline included recommendations regarding _____alcohol_____.

<u>SUMMING UP</u>

<u>Review text</u>

<u>SELF STUDY</u>

Check with instructor if "Self Study" (Appendix Q in textbook) will be assigned at this time.

Forms for completing Self Study assignments are at the end of this book.

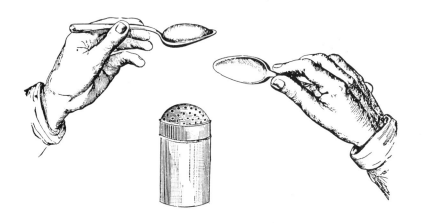

ANSWERS

1. eat
2. molecules, organs
3. replaced, nutrients, energy
4. 120, three
5. eaten
6. nutrients, nutrients
7. maintenance
8. food
9. Carbohydrate, fat, protein, vitamins, minerals, water
10. water
11. additives, pollutants
12. gas, ash
13. carbon
14. organic
15. minerals, water
16. fat, protein, carbohydrate
17. oxidized
18. mechanical
19. nutrients, energy
20. vitamins, minerals
21. kcalories
22. gram, one
23. kilojoules
24. energy
25. energy
26. carbohydrate, fat
27. energy
28. 100, 5
29. cups
30. organic, 15
31. destructible
32. light
33. fat
34. inorganic, 21
35. inorganic
36. indestructible

37. acid-base
38. water
39. ten
40. energy
41. lungs
42. Adequacy, Balance, Calorie control, and Variety
43. Protein foods, calcium-rich foods, fruits and vegetables, whole grain cereals or breads
44. sugar, fat
45. flexible, do not
46. E
47. legumes, 3/4 cup, 3 oz.
48. whole grain, E
49. 2,200, adequacy
50. legumes
51. two, lacto-ovo, vegan, B
52. nutrient density
53. nutritious foods
54. necessary, kcalories
55. optimal
56. foundation foods, dense, grains
57. six, milk, vegetable, fruit.
58. meat
59. 4, 9, 4.
60. milk, fat
61. corn, lima beans
62. exchange list
63. dietary, Canada
64. Recommended Dietary Allowances
65. 12
66. five
67. scientific, requirements
68. different
69. individual
70. restoration
71. mean
72. carbohydrate, fat
73. food labels
74. RDA, man
75. iron
76. data
77. Agriculture
78. Health
79. all people
80. higher, lower
81. higher
82. higher, high
83. dietary intake
84. nutrient

85.   subclinical
86.   deficiencies
87.   healthy, normally
88.   examination
89.   laboratory
90.   growth, swelling
91.   recommendations
92.   Canadians
93.   United States
94.   Americans
95.   disagreement
96.   salt
97.   complex
98.   nutrients, foods
99.   disbanded
100. USDA
101. alcohol

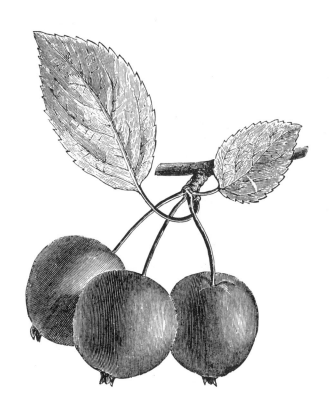

HIGHLIGHT 1A: NATURAL FOODS

1. The term ___organic___ has two meanings.

2. Rodale's definition of an organic food is " a food grown with manure or compost, unsprayed with pesticides, and processed without the use of ___food___ ___additives___ ."

3. As defined by chemists, the term <u>organic</u> merely means "containing atoms of ___carbon___ ."

4. The word ___organic___ on a food label usually conveys the Rodale meaning. Another word that means almost the same is " ___natural___ ."

5. "Health foods" include both " ___organic___ " and "natural" foods.

6. They include conventional foods which have been subjected to less processing, such as whole-grain flours, and ___less___ conventional foods such as brewer's yeast and wheat germ.

7. " ___Health___ ___food___ " is usually a misleading term implying unusual power to promote health. Further, this term has no legal ___definition___ .

Cons of Health Foods

8. When the users of health foods are observed, what they are really trying to buy is ___peace___ of mind.

9. "Health foods" can cost as much as ___50___ percent or more than comparable grocery-store items.

10. Almost ___100___ million dollars a year is spent on herbal products, much of it by mail.

11. Herbal preparations can contain ___natural___ toxins.

12. _Herbal_ _tease_ can even cause food poisoning symptoms.

13. Products sold under the label "health" may not be so healthy after all. As of the Fall of 1979, _700_ different plants had been reported to cause deaths or serious illnesses and none were caused by the consumption of legally-permitted levels of artificial additives in processed foods.

14. Honey should probably not be fed to _infant_ under one year of age.

15. Terms such as "health food," "natural," and "organic" should be _prohibited_ from use on labels.

16. Some health-food store operators are _dishonest_ , and some sellers label their products organic just to be able to raise the price.

Pros of Organic Farming

17. Organic foods are grown in soil that is fertilized only with natural _waste_ material.

18. Chemical fertilizers are good if they provide the plant with a "balanced _diet_ . "

19. The ultimate chemical composition achieved by a plant depends on the _genetic_ _program_ it has received from its seeds.

20. If the fertilizer is inadequate, then the crop yield will be _less_ , but what plants there are will be of the usual composition.

21. An exception to this relates to _minerals_ .

22. Plants grown in soil lacking iodine will produce _iodine_ - _poor_ fruits and vegetables.

23. Natural fertilizers affect the _structure_ of the soil.

24. The most significant difference between organic and conventional farming may be to the _ecology_ ; organic farming conserves _energy_ and doesn't pollute.

17

25. Conventional agriculture consumes vast amounts of __energy__ and produces half of the solid waste the United States generates each year.

26. Generally speaking, the more a food resembles the original, farm-grown produce, the more __nutritious__ it is likely to be.

27. Nutrients are lost and empty kcalorie additions like sugar, salt, and __fat__ are added during processing.

28. A potato and an apple don't have to be labeled natural, they only have to __be__ natural.

29. Health-food stores often ignore the principle of __nutrient__ __density__.

30. It is __possible__ (possible/impossible) to obtain nutritious foods by making educated __choices__ in the grocery store.

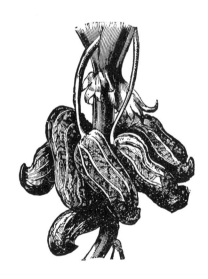

ANSWERS

1. organic
2. food additives
3. carbon
4. organic, natural.
5. organic
6. less
7. Health food, definition
8. peace
9. 50
10. 100
11. natural
12. Herbal teas
13. 700
14. infants
15. prohibited
16. dishonest
17. waste
18. diet
19. genetic program
20. less
21. minerals
22. iodine-poor
23. structure
24. ecology, energy
25. energy
26. nutritious
27. fat
28. be
29. nutrient density
30. possible, choices

HIGHLIGHT 1B: VITAMIN SUPPLEMENTS

1. All substances are poison. The right dose differentiates a poison and a ____remedy____.

2. Approximately ____two-thirds____ of our citizens use vitamin pills.

3. Many people view a single vitamin pill every day as "nutritional ____insurance____."

4. Even if unnecessary, this practice is not ____harmful____.

5. Pills and powders do not substitute for ____food____.

6. Nutritional faddism is born of inadequate ____knowledge____.

Nutritional Individuality

7. There are normal ____variation____ between individuals, but they are not large.

8. Nutrient requirements are determined by genetic patterns, stress, or various ____illnesses____.

How Vitamins are Promoted

9. A lot of vitamins are sold by exaggerating the idea of ____subclinical____ deficiency.

10. The body cannot tell whether a vitamin in the bloodstream came from an organically grown product or from a ____chemists____ laboratory.

11. There may be ____fringe____ benefits to eating nutrients in a natural food instead of a purified preparation.

Minerals: Even More Dangerous

12. Cell salts are mineral preparations prepared from living, __health__ __cells__ .

13. Hair analysis __has not__ (has/has not) been found appropriate for general nutritional evaluation.

14. If your kcalorie intake is below 1,500 kcalories a day, then it is appropriate to take a vitamin-mineral __supplement__ .

15. If your eating is very irregular, a __vitamin__ - __minerals__ supplement is called for.

16. The most risky supplements are vitamin __A__ and D capsules, minerals, and potassium __chloride__ .

17. Powdered bone (bonemeal) has been found to contain high levels of __lead__ .

18. People taking kelp tablets regularly may show raised urinary concentrations of __arsenic__ .

19. Toxicity is also possible with vitamins __C__ and __E__ .

20. Spirulina may make vitamin __B__ less available to the body.

21. Nutritional yeast is a __good__ source of protein, B-vitamins, and iron.

22. Wheat germ, granola, and powdered skim milk are __nutritious__ foods.

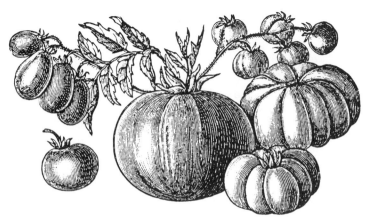

ANSWERS

1. remedy
2. two-thirds
3. insurance
4. harmful
5. food
6. knowledge
7. variations
8. illnesses
9. subclinical
10. chemist's
11. fringe
12. healthy cells
13. has not
14. supplement
15. vitamin-mineral
16. A, chloride
17. lead
18. arsenic
19. C, E
20. B
21. good
22. nutritious

SELF TEST

1. You are a collection of _____ that move.
    a. molecules
    b. nutrients
    c. organic compounds
    d. inorganic compounds

2. Your oldest blood cell is only _____ days
    old.
    a. 30
    b. 300
    c. 120
    d. 1,200

3. The entire lining of your digestive tract is renewed every
    _____ days.
    a. 2
    b. 3
    c. 15
    d. 150

4. Nutritive material taken into the body to keep it alive is
    called:
    a. digestive material.
    b. carbohydrates.
    c. protein.
    d. food.

5. A substance obtained from food and used in the body to
    promote growth, maintenance, and/or repair is called:
    a. a nutrient.
    b. fat.
    c. an organic compound.
    d. an inorganic compound.

6. A substance the body cannot make and must obtain from food
    is called:
    a.   a nutrient.
    b.   an essential nutrient.
    c.   a maintenance substance.
    d.   a vitamin.

7. An organic compound is one that:
    a.   contains carbon atoms.
    b.   is more nutritious.
    c.   is free of chemical additives.
    d.   is natural.

8. The organic nutrients are:
    a.   carbohydrate and fat.
    b.   protein and vitamins.
    c.   minerals and water.
    d.   a and b.
    e.   b and c.

9. A reaction in which atoms from a molecule are combined with
    oxygen, usually with the release of energy, is called:
    a.   oxidation.
    b.   metabolism.
    c.   reduction.

10. The set of processes by which nutrients are rearranged into
    body structures, or broken down to yield energy, is called:
    a.   oxidation.
    b.   metabolism.
    c.   reduction.
    d.   absorption.

11. Food energy is measured in:
    a.   calories.
    b.   kcalories.
    c.   kilojoules.
    d.   all of the above.
    e.   none of the above.

12. The amount of heat necessary to raise the temperature of a
    gram of water one degree Centigrade is technically known as
    a:
    a.   gram.
    b.   kilogram.
    c.   calorie.
    d.   milliliter.

13. The weight of a serving of most vegetables, or a half cup
    of milk or juice, is roughly:
    a. 50 grams.
    b. 100 grams.
    c. 5 grams.
    d. 10 grams.

14. Vitamins are:
    a. indestructible.
    b. destructible.
    c. ionic.
    d. inorganic molecules.

15. The most important division of vitamins into two classes in
    the division between_____and_____vitamins.
    a. organic, and inorganic
    b. synthetic, and natural
    c. water-soluble, fat-soluble

16. Minerals are:
    a. inorganic.
    b. organic.
    c. destructible.
    d. none of the above

17. If a person follows all the rules of the "Basic Four,
    "nutritional adequacy will be guaranteed.
    a. True
    b. False

18. The Modified Four Food Group Plan suggests:
    a. two servings legumes and/or nuts.
    b. using whole-grain, not enriched, products.
    c. adding one serving of fat or oil.
    d. use 3-oz potions of meat, fish or poultry.
    e. all of the above.

19. A lacto-ovo-vegetarian:
    a. uses milk and eggs.
    b. uses milk but not eggs.
    c. eats vegetables; no milk, meat, or eggs.
    d. uses cheese, eggs, and vegetables.

20. The exchange system has _____ lists of foods.
    a. one
    b. three
    c. four
    d. five
    e. six

21.   The exchange system controls intakes of:
  a.   kcalories, fat, protein, and carbohydrate.
  b.   fat, protein, and carbohydrate.
  c.   vitamins and minerals.
  d.   types of food eaten.
  e.   kcalories, carbohydrate, and protein.

22.   If 10 potato chips have absorbed 8 grams of fat during
      frying, how many kcalories have been added to them?
      a.   80   b.   90   c.   72   d.   108

23.   If a slice of bread contains 15 grams carbohydrate, and 2
      grams protein, and no fat, about how many kcalories are in
      the bread?
      a.   50   b.   60   c.   70   d.   80   e.   90

24.   Which statement is not true about the RDAs?
      a.   They are published by the government
      b.   They are based on available scientific evidence
      c.   They are minimum requirements for healthy persons only
      d.   They take into account the range within which most
           healthy persons' intakes of nutrients probably
           should be.

25.   A laboratory study in which a person is fed a controlled
      diet and the intake and excretion of a nutrient are
      measured is called:
      a.   a balance study.
      b.   a double-blind experiment.
      c.   a nutrition test.
      d.   a lab volunteer.

26.   No RDA is set for _____ or _____ .
      a.   energy, calories
      b.   carbohydrate, fat
      c.   infants, children under 6

27.   The term _____ appears on food labels.
      a.   U.S.   RDA
      b.   RDA
      c.   nutritional analysis
      d.   nutrition information

28. The seventh of the <u>Dietary guidelines for Americans</u> is a
     recommendation regarding:
     a. fat.
     b. salt.
     c. whole grains.
     d. alcohol.
     e. kcalories.

29. The final excretory products of the oxidation of protein,
     fat, or carbohydrate are:
     a. carbon dioxide and water.
     b. urea and uric acid.
     c. waste matter from the colon.
     d. none of the above.

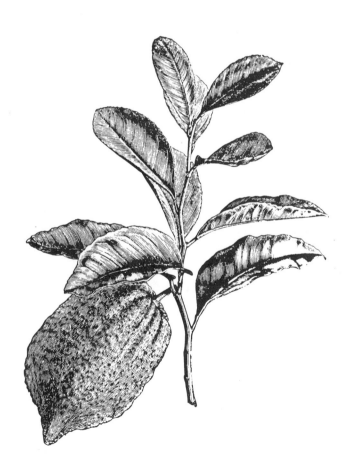

ANSWERS

1.   a
2.   c
3.   b
4.   d
5.   a
6.   b
7.   a
8.   d
9.   a
10.   b
11.   d
12.   c
13.   b
14.   b
15.   c
16.   a
17.   b
18.   e
19.   a
20.   e
21.   a
22.   c
23.   c
24.   c
25.   a
26.   b
27.   a
28.   b
29.   a

RECIPES YOU CAN TRY...

VERSATILE BEANS AND LEGUMES

Now that you have been introduced to the idea of using more beans and legumes in your diet, here is some important information, and ideas for inexpensive main dishes using them.

Recipes which use beans are highly adaptable; in other words, you can substitute most any bean for the bean the recipe calls for. This goes for salads, soups, main dishes--even chili bean recipes.

TIMETABLE FOR COOKING DRY BEANS

1 cup dry beans (soaked)	Simmering time in saucepan	Pressure-cooking time Minutes at 15 pounds pressure*
Black beans	2 hours	35
Black-eyed beans (peas, cowpeas)	25 to 30 minutes	10
Garbanzo beans (chick peas)	2 to 2-1/4 hours	40
Great Northern beans	1 to 1-1/2 hours	30
Kidney beans	1-1/2 hours	30
Lima beans, large	1 hour	30
Lima beans, small	45 minutes	25
Pea (navy) beans	1-1/2 hours	30
Pink beans	2 hours	30
Red beans	2 hours	30
Soybeans	3 to 3-1/2 hours	40

In slow-cooker, cook soaked beans on low heat about 8 hours or until tender.

---

*NOTE: Be careful not to fill pressure saucepan more than half full because foaming can clog vent and blow gasket.

RECIPES YOU CAN TRY...

DRIED BEAN PATTIES

Grind and mash:
     2 cups cooked dried beans: soy, lima, navy
Add to them:
     1 chopped onion
     1/4 cup chopped parsley
Beat and add:
     1 egg
     1/4 tsp pepper
     1 tsp salt

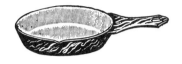

Shape these ingredients into balls and flatten. Dip into flour.
Chill the patties for 1 hour or more. Heat 1 or 2 tbsp butter,
margarine, or oil in a frying pan. Saute the patties on each
side until browned. Serve with melted cheese or barbecue sauce.
Makes six servings.

LENTILS CREOLE

1 cup dried lentils
1 tsp salt
2 tbsp butter or margarine
2 sweet peppers, minced
1 onion, chopped

2 cups canned tomatoes
1/4 tsp pepper
1 tsp sugar
cooked rice or noodles

1) Cover the lentils with boiling water and soak for
     15 minutes
2) Then boil in salted water about 1 hour and drain.
3) Melt the butter in a saucepan: add green peppers and
     onions. Cook slowly until the butter browns.
4) Add the tomatoes, pepper, and sugar to the lentils and
     simmer 30 to 40 minutes.
5) Serve over rice or noodles. Makes four servings.

BULGUR RECIPES

Bulgur, a precooked, cracked wheat, selected recently by the U.S.
government for export to needy countries, resembles brown rice.
It can be used in any way that rice is used. Bulgur requires very
little cooking.

Bulgur pilaf is an alternative to potatoes. It can be used in
main dishes or added to various soups. It is high in available
protein and fiber, and contains important B vitamins.

30

To cook bulgur:

1 cup bulgur wheat, uncooked
2 cups water
1 tsp salt

In a pan, combine bulgur wheat, water, and salt; bring to a boil, stir, cover, and simmer 10 to 15 minutes or until tender and liquid is absorbed.

SPINACH CASSEROLE

3/4 cup raw bulgur, cooked
1/2 cup grated cheddar cheese
1 lb fresh spinach, chopped
2 eggs, beaten

2 tbsp parsley, chopped
1/2 tsp salt
1/4 tsp pepper
2 tbsp wheat germ
1 tbsp melted butter

Mix together the cooked bulgur, and cheese. Mix the eggs, parsley, salt, and pepper. Combine the two mixtures together, and stir in the raw spinach. Pour into an oiled casserole. Top with wheat germ which has been mixed with the melted butter. Bake in a 350° oven for 35 minutes.

BULGUR PILAF

2 tbsp oil
1 tbsp onion, chopped
1 cup bulgur
Chopped parsley for garnish

2 cups water or chicken or
    beef stock
1/2 tsp. salt
dash of pepper

Put oil in skillet; add onion and saute until almost tender (about 8 minutes). Add bulgur and cook until golden. Add stock or water and seasonings. Cover and bring to a boil; reduce heat and simmer 15 minutes. Garnish with chopped parsley and serve. (4 servings)

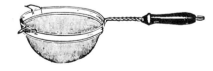

CHAPTER 2

The Carbohydrates: Sugar, Starch, and Fiber

YOU WILL LEARN...

1. The importance of your blood sugar level--which affects the way you think, act, and feel.

2. How the blood glucose level is maintained.

3. How sugar looks to a chemist and what it is made of.

4. How carbohydrates are taken apart.

5. How complex carbohydrates look to a chemist.

6. The role of fiber is in the diet and how it is different from other carbohydrates.

7. How much carbohydrate you need in your diet and how you get it from food.

8. Which exchange lists include carbohydrate?

9. To differentiate between alternative sweeteners and artificial sweeteners.

HIGHLIGHT 2: SUGAR STANDS ACCUSED

13. What the six main arguments against sugar are.

14. What course you might choose for yourself after reading the evidence.

CARBOHYDRATES: SUGAR, STARCH, AND FIBER

1. You can feel really good only when your _____ _____ level is right.

2. The simple sugar called _____ is often called blood sugar, because it is the principal carbohydrate found in the blood of mammals.

3. The status of your blood sugar determines how you think, act, and feel because the cells of your _____ and _____ system normally depend on this sugar to facilitate their energy metabolism.

4. No energy source other than _____ is normally utilized by the brain and nerves.

5. When there is too <u>little</u> glucose in the blood we call it _____. Symptoms can include weakness, trembling, anxiety, dizziness, or nausea.

6. Similar symptoms can be caused by _____ deprivation of the brain, extreme anxiety, or even multiple sclerosis.

THE CONSTANCY OF THE BLOOD GLUCOSE LEVEL

7. The normal fasting blood glucose concentration range is _____ mg/100 ml. Hunger is usually experienced at the low end of the normal range, _____ mg/100 ml. A milligram (mg) is _____ of a gram.

8. It is important that the blood glucose level should not rise too high and the body protects itself against this eventuality. The first organ to respond to raised blood glucose is the _____ which detects the excess and sends out a message.

9. The _____, and _____ cells receive
    the message, remove the glucose from the blood, and store
    it. The liver cells also convert it to _____ and make
    it ready for transport to the _____ cells.

10. The hormone excreted by the pancreas is called _____.
    The special cells that secrete insulin are called
    _____ cells.

11. Most cells use glucose for energy right away, but the
    _____ and _____ cells have the ability to store it for
    later use. The storage form of glucose is called
    _____

12. Fat cells conserve the energy of glucose in the form of
    _____.

13. Before you eat again, if your brain or other body cells
    need glucose it will be supplied from _____, but only
    from the liver, not from the muscles.

14. A hormone that can call glucose out of the liver cells in
    times of stress is _____. At ordinary times other
    hormones such as _____ insure that glucose be
    brought out of storage in the liver. Glucagon is produced
    by the _____ cells of the pancreas.

15. Muscle _____ is used primarily within the muscle
    cells themselves, but can be broken down to an intermediate
    product, _____.

16. Learning to maintain your own blood sugar at the optimum
    level is most important if you are to think, act, and feel
    your best.

    a. When you are hungry, you should eat without waiting
        until you are famished.

    b. You should eat balanced meals including
        some _____ and _____ as well as complex
        carbohydrate.

17. Diabetes is a disease in which raised blood sugar is not
    withdrawn into cells. Instead, the glucose _____
    into the urine. Excessive _____ and _____
    are symptoms of this defect in carbohydrate metabolism.

18. Diabetes is present in about _____ out of every
    _____ families in the United States and Canada.

THE CHEMIST'S VIEW OF SUGARS

Glucose

19. A chemist views a glucose molecule as a compound composed of _____ atoms: ____ carbons, _____ hydrogens, and _____ oxygens. Thus the chemical formula for glucose is: _____.

20. Each type of atom has a characteristic amount of energy for forming chemical _____ with other atoms.

21. A carbon atom can form _____ (bond/bonds).

22. An oxygen atom can form _____ (bond/bonds).

23. A hydrogen atom forms _____ bond.

24. One way to represent the number of bonds associated with each type of atom is to use _____ radiating from the letters.

25. The bonds of the carbon atom are represented by showing _____ lines radiating from each –C–.

26. The bonds of an oxygen atom are represented by _____ lines.

27. The bond of a hydrogen atom is represented by _____ line.

28. –C– represents the bonds of a _____ atom.

29. –O– represents the bonds of a _____ atom.

30. H– represents the bonds of a _____ atom.

31. In the simplest terms, you can build many things out of only these three elements--like a child's set of "tinker toys"--as long as the _____ requirements are met.

32. Complete the chemical structure of _____ alcohol:

    H – C --C-- O – H

33. ALL carbohydrates are composed at least partly of _____ and other C-H-O compounds very much like glucose in structure.

34.   Glucose and other C-H-O compounds come in three main sizes:

    a.   _____ molecules like glucose itself.
    b.   _____ of glucose molecules bonded together.
    c.   Chains.

35.   The chemist's terms for these three types of carbohydrates are:

    a.   Monosaccharides   b.   Disaccharides
    c.   _____

36.   Understanding bonding requirements, and the ways that glucose units can be put together enables you to understand the differences between sugars, and starches, and how they are handled by the body.

    a.   The sugars, also known as the simple carbohydrates, are the _____ and _____. Sucrose, or table sugar, is a _____.

    b.   Complex carbohydrates such as starch, glycogen, and some fibers are the _____.

37.   Monosaccharides include _____, _____, and _____.

38.   Disaccharides include _____ _____ and _____

39.   Mono- and disaccharides are simple carbohydrates, also called the _____.

Making and Breaking Pairs: Chemical Reactions

40.   When a disaccharide is formed from two monosaccharides, a chemical reaction known as a _____ reaction takes place.

41.   In a condensation reaction, something is taken away--thus condensed. A simple definition of condensation would be "a chemical reaction in which two reactants combine to yield a major product, with the elimination of _____ or a similar small molecule."

42. More technically, you could say that in a condensation reaction a _____ atom is removed from one monosaccharide and an oxygen hydrogen (OH) group is removed from the other, leaving the two molecules bonded by a single -O-.

43. When a disaccharide is taken apart to form two monosaccharides again, as for example during digestion in the human body, a molecule of water participates in the reaction, with the H- being added to one, and the -O-H to the other monosaccharide, to reform the original structures. This reaction is called a _____ reaction.

44. All of the carbohydrates are put together and taken apart by _____ and _____ reactions.

45. The facilitators of condensation and hydrolysis reactions are _____.

46. An enzyme is a giant molecule which provides a surface on which other molecules may come together and _____ with each other.

47. The making and _____ of chemical bonds tells the whole story of growth, maintenance, and change in living creatures. The _____ that facilitate these reactions are indispensable to life.

THE SUGARS

48. Virtually all our energy comes from the food we eat, about half from carbohydrate and half from _____ and _____.

49. One of the principal roles of carbohydrate in the diet is to supply energy in the form of _____ glucose.

50. The six common sugars found in food--the mono- and disaccharides--are glucose, fructose, _____; sucrose, lactose, and _____.

51. Other sugars used in special dietary products, made from sugar alcohols, are maltitol, mannitol, xylitol, and _____.

52. _____ is not expecially sweet tasting, but it can be absorbed directly into the bloodstream.

53. Fruit sugar is called _____.

54. The sweetest of all the sugars is _____.

55. In the body, the effect of fructose is very similar to the effect of _____.

56. The sweet taste we experience comes from the arrangement of C - H - O atoms stimulating certain receptors in the tongue. These arrangements_____(can/cannot)be duplicated artificially.

57. Saccharin, cyclamate, and aspartame are examples of _____ or _____ sweeteners.

58. Galactose is seldom found free in nature but occurs as part of the disaccharide _____.

59. The chemical formula for the hexoses--glucose, fructose and galactose-- is: _____.

60. A molecule shared in common by all three disaccharides is _____.

61. The sweet taste of sucrose comes from _____.

62. Lactose is the principal carbohydrate found in _____.

63. A human baby is born with the digestive _____ necessary to hydrolyze lactose into its two monosaccharide parts, glucose, and _____.

64. Galactose is converted to glucose in the liver, so each molecule of lactose yields two molecules of glucose to supply energy for a baby's growth and activity; babies can digest _____ at birth, but they don't develop the ability to digest _____ until they are several months old.

65. If you lose the ability to digest lactose, you are said to be _____ _____.

66. Lactose intolerance, whether inherited or acquired, is due to failure to produce the _____ lactose.

67. The disaccharide made of two glucose units, sometimes known as malt sugar, is called _____.

68.   The malt found in beer, or in the seeds of grains, is
      called _____.

THE CHEMIST'S VIEW OF COMPLEX CARBOHYDRATES

69.   Polysaccharides are composed almost entirely of
      _____ units strung together in long branched
      chains.

70.   A plant polysaccharide composed of glucose and digestible
      by humans is called _____.

71.   All _____ foods are in fact plant foods. In making
      starch, the plant was actually preparing for its own first
      growth.

72.   Wheat, rice, corn, millet, rye, barley, and oats are
      examples of _____ _____.

73.   A second important source of starch, also known as
      "legumes," is the _____ and pea family. Examples
      include pinto beans, lima beans, garbanzo beans, cowpeas,
      yellow and green dried peas, and soybeans.

74.   A third major source of starch is _____ such as
      potato, yam, and cassava.

75.   When you eat starchy foods, starch molecules are taken
      apart by _____ in your mouth and intestine. The
      enzymes _____ the starch into _____ units
      which are absorbed from the intestinal wall into the blood.

76.   Starch can be broken down to shorter chains of glucose
      units called _____, which can be used commercially as
      thickening agents in foods.

77.   The kind of starch stored in the liver and muscle of animals
      is called _____.

THE FIBERS
Cellulose

78.   Cellulose, like starch, is found abundantly in plants and
      has long chains of glucose units. However, the _____
      are different and humans have no enzymes to release the
      energy from cellulose.

79. Cellulose, does, however, provide _____ in our diet, which is important to human nutrition.

80. Three carbohydrates provide indigestible residue, and so are classified as fiber. They are: pectin, cellulose, and _____.

81. An example of an indigestible noncarbohydrate is _____.

82. Still others are gums and mucilages often used as thickening agents in _____ foods.

83. Food fiber_____(is/is not) calorie-free.

84. Dietary fiber may:

    a. Speed up the passage of foods through the digestive tract.
    b. Reduce cholesterol level by inhibiting reabsorption of bile acids.
    c. Bind carcinogens and prevent their absorption.
    d. Protect against diverticulitis.
    e. Promote weight_____ (loss/gain).

85. A high-fiber diet helps manage diabetes, reducing the need for_____.

86. The fiber of _____ has a greater cholesterol-lowering effect than the fiber of _____.

87. The best stool-softening fiber is _____.

88. The typical Western diet is _____ (low/high) in fiber.

89. Food processing enhances the insulin response to a food even when no _____ is removed.

90. The presence of too much insulin in the blood is associated with _____ and _____ disease as well as with diabetes.

91. High-fiber diets involve a significant reduction in _____ and _____ containing foods.

92. Fiber-rich foods help in weight control because they satisfy _____ as well as having fewer kcalories than refined foods.

93. Fiber also helps to protect against _____ of the colon and rectum.

Too Much Fiber

94. Too much bulk in the diet could cause too great a decrease in intakes of both _____ and _____.

95. One trace mineral whose absorption could be reduced by consuming too much fiber is _____.

96. The substance in food called _____ acid could cause losses of zinc, iron, calcium, copper, and magnesium.

97. Phytic acid is found in the husks of grains, legumes, and seeds, but is destroyed by _____.

Estimating Fiber Amounts in Foods .

98. Crude fiber is what remains in the laboratory after a food is digested with _____ and bases.

99. Dietary fiber is what remains from food after _____ in the body.

100. _____ fiber constitutes a larger residue than _____ fiber.

101. Since most fiber contents of foods are reported as crude fiber, it is well to remember that _____ g of crude fiber equals about _____ g of dietary fiber.

How Much Fiber Is Enough?

102. What is the RDA for fiber? _____.

103. An average of _____ grams of crude fiber daily is thought to be sufficient for body needs.

104. The African studies that suggested a beneficial effect of fiber were based on levels as high as _____ grams.

105. The best way to add fiber to your diet is to increase your use of fruits, vegetables, _____ and nuts.

CHAPTER 2: THE CARBOHYDRATES SUGAR, STARCH AND FIBER

THE CARBOHYDRATES IN FOODS

106.   The "Protein-sparing effect" of carbohydrate means that if
        you don't eat carbohydrate your body devours its own
        _____ to generate glucose.

107.   Most experts seem to agree that you need somewhere around
        100 to 300 grams of _____ per day.

108.   Carbohydrates have _____ kcal/gram. Later you will
        learn that protein has 4 kcal/gram and fat has 9 kcal/gram.
        You can see the fallacy of the idea that starch is "more
        fattening" than meat.

109.   If you have trouble understanding the "exchange lists"
        described in Chapter 1, think of them as "substitution
        lists." Foods are grouped so that the carbohydrate
        contents of individual items within a group are _____

110.   Carbohydrate is found in _____ of the six types of foods
        in the exchange system.

111.   To estimate carbohydrate value you need to memorize four
        exchange-system values: Milk, _____; Bread, _____; Fruit,
        _____; Vegetable, _____; and "Sugar," _____.

112.   Remember that when you figure the GRAMS of carbohydrate you
        have to multiply by ____ to figure the kcalories.

113.   A 12-ounce can of a sugary carbonated beverage contains
        about 9 tsp sugar, or ____ g carbohydrate and _____
        kcalories.

Alternative Sweeteners

114.   Review: Sugar alcohols used as alternative sweeteners
        include _____, maltitol, _____, and xylitol.

115.   Mannitol is less _____ than sucrose and tends to cause
        diarrhea.

116.   Sorbitol is much used for sugar-free gums and candies but
        it is only _____ as sweet as sucrose so twice as many
        kcalories are present. Fortunately it has little or no
        effect on _____ glucose, so people with diabetes may
        benefit from its use.

117.   xylitol helps prevent _____ _____ but may
        cause tumors in animals.

118.   The sugar alcohols contain as many calories as sucrose but the body handles them _____.

119.   Fructose is _____ as sweet as sucrose and does not stimulate insulin secretion, but it does contain _____ kcal/g.

120.   Aspartame, cyclamate, and _____ are the most popular artificial sweeteners in use today.

121.   Aspartame is _____ times sweeter than sucrose. It is blended with lactose and sold as "Equal." It cannot be used for cooking and baking, but when unheated has no bitter _____.

122.   Cyclamate is a _____ kcalorie sweetener, now banned in the United States.

123.   Saccharin is a _____ kcalorie sweetener, now banned in Canada.

Fiber

124.   Table 2-4 shows that fruits, vegetables, and breads and cereals have about _____ grams of fiber per serving.

125.   The advertisers that tell us that a candy bar and a cola beverage are the best sources for "quick energy" are _____.

SUMMING UP

126.   At least _____ of our food energy is derived from carbohydrate.

127.   All of the monosaccharides share the same chemical formula: _____.

128.   Each of the three disaccharides contains a molecule of _____ paired with either fructose, galacose, or another _____.

129.   The energy in concentrated sweets such as cakes and candy comes from _____.

130.   We store starch in our bodies only in the form of _____.

131. Carbohydrates contain _____ kcalories per gram. There are 5 grams of carbohydrate in a teaspoon of sugar and there are _____kcalories.

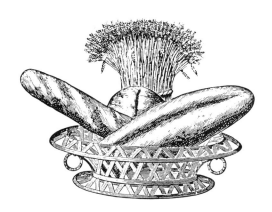

ANSWERS

1. blood sugar
2. glucose
3. brain, nervous
4. glucose
5. hypoglycemia
6. oxygen
7. 80-120; 60 or 70; 1/1,000
8. pancreas
9. liver, muscle, fat, adipose
10. insulin, beta
11. liver, muscle, glycogen
12. fat
13. glycogen
14. epinephrine; glucagon, alpha
15. glycogen, lactate
16. protein, fat
17. "spills", hunger, thirst
18. one, four
19. 24, 6, 12, 6; $C_6H_{12}O_6$
20. bonds
21. 4
22. 2
23. 1
24. lines
25. 4
26. 2
27. 1
28. carbon
29. oxygen
30. hydrogen
31. bonding
32. ethyl
33. glucose
34. Single, Pairs
35. polysaccharides

36. a. monosaccharides, disaccharides ,disaccharide
    b. polysaccharides
37. glucose, fructose, galactose
38. sucrose, lactose, maltose
39. sugars
40. condensation
41. water
42. hydrogen
43. hydrolysis
44. condensation, hydrolysis
45. enzymes
46. react
47. breaking, emzymes
48. protein, fat
49. blood
50. galactose, maltose
51. sorbitol
52. Glucose
53. fructose
54. fructose
55. glucose
56. can
57. artificial, non-nutritive
58. lactose
59. $C_6H_{12}O_6$
60. glucose
61. fructose
62. milk
63. enzymes, galactose
64. lactose, starch
65. lactose intolerant
66. enzyme
67. maltose
68. maltose
69. glucose
70. starch
71. starchy
72. staple grains
73. bean
74. tubers
75. enzymes, hydrolyze, glucose
76. dextrins
77. glycogen
78. bonds
79. fiber
80. hemicellulose
81. lignin
82. prepared
83. is not

CHAPTER 2 : ANSWERS

84. loss
85. insulin
86. apples, wheat
87. bran
88. low
89. fiber
90. obesity, heart
91. fat, protein
92. hunger
93. cancer
94. nutrients, kcalories
95. iron
96. phytic
97. heat
98. acids
99. digestion
100. dietary, crude
101. 1,2-3
102. There is none
103. 4-7
104. 25
105. whole grains
106. protein
107. carbohydrate
108. 4
109. similar
110. 4
111. 12, 15, 10, 5, 5
112. 4
113. 45, 180
114. mannitol, sorbitol
115. sweet
116. half, blood
117. dental caries
118. differently
119. twice, 4
120. saccharin
121. 200, aftertaste
122. zero
123. zero
124. two
125. wrong
126. half
127. $C_6H_{12}O_6$
128. glucose, glucose
129. sucrose
130. glycogen
131. 4, 20

SUGAR STANDS ACCUSED

1. Briefly, six arguments against sugar will be analyzed:
    1. Concentrated sugar is new in the human diet.
    2. Sugar in the diet displaces other nutrients.
    3. If you eat nutrients + sugar, you get fat.
    4. Excess sugar may stress the pancreas.
    5. Sugar may lead to heart disease.
    6. Sugar also causes _____ _____.

Evidence

2. We do require _____ in our diet but the body has no
    need for _____ itself.

3. Sugar consumption in the United States has increased from
    _____ pounds per person per year in 1820 to over
    _____ pounds in the 1970s. In Canada it is now between
    _____ and _____ pounds per person per year.

4. In the present, over_____percent of the kcalories in our
    diet come from sugars and visible fats, and sugar is
    today's leading additive.

5. Of the 100-plus pounds of sugar that we eat in a year,
    _____ some pounds are already added to foods during
    processing.

6. Children with kidney disease might be an exception to the
    rule that sugar should be avoided because it helps them
    _____.

7. White sugar, after digestion, yields a fifty-fifty mixture
    of glucose and _____.

8. As such, the glucose from sugar is the same as the glucose
    from _____.

9. Starch comes in foods with other nutrients, while sugar can be termed an _____ _____ food.

10. Whether you can afford to eat sugar depends on how many kcalories you have to _____ altogether.

11. Sugar can clearly cause malnutrition if it is substituted for _____ dense foods.

12. Some of the effects of sugar on behavior may be due to poor _____.

13. Excess kcalories from any energy nutrient, even _____, are stored in body fat.

14. Sugar _____ (is/is not) the sole cause.

15. Where sugar intake increases, _____ _____ decreases.

16. Diabetes is not one, but _____ disorders.

17. The predominant type is non-insulin-dependent diabetes. Insulin-dependent diabetes is less common. Another type is caused by _____ deficiency.

18. Wherever starch (or the fiber or the chromium that goes with it) is a major part of the diet, diabetes is _____.

19. In most of the world, when sugar consumption has increased, a profound increase--by as much as _____ fold--in the incidence of diabetes has also occurred.

20. Diabetes can be induced in experimental animals by feeding them diets high in fat, protein, or _____ and can be reduced by _____ total food intake.

21. However, diets very high in sugar can cause the disease even if the animals do not become _____.

22. An early symptom of diabetes is excessive _____.

23. Both weight _____ and avoidance of _____ are recommended for the potential diabetic.

24. Although high sugar correlates with increased blood fat levels and deaths from heart disease, the deaths are associated more closely with _____ than with sugar intake.

25. Moderate amounts of sugar _____ (do/do not) affect the disease process of atherosclerosis.

26. Another name for atherosclerosis is _____ of the _____.

27. Dental caries affects nearly _____.

28. Dental caries are actually caused by the _____ of bacterial growth in the mouth.

29. Food for the bacteria could be provided by either sugar or _____.

30. A sweetened beverage might actually cause less decay than raisins or _____.

31. A statement of the amount of dental decay a food would produce would be a _____ index for the food.

32. Damage from sugar to the tooth surface is maximal within the first _____ minutes after the first contact.

33. Some people _____ (may/may not) be resistant to cavities.

Conclusion

34. Honey is clearly _____ (better/worse/the same) as sugar.

35. An "instant breakfast" is a _____ (good/poor) replacement for a balanced meal.

36. Sugar is "bad" for the dieter, not because it is _____ but because it displaces nutritious foods.

37. Is sugar "bad" for you? _____ (yes/no/maybe).

38. Is sugar "good" for you? _____ (yes/no/maybe).

39. Should we switch to saccharin? _____ (yes/no/maybe).

40. Should we switch to aspartame? _____ (yes/no/maybe).

41. The best course for most to follow is probably
     _____.

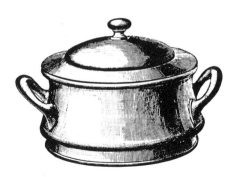

ANSWERS

1. dental caries
2. carbohydrate, sugar
3. 20,100, 87, 98
4. 33
5. 70
6. grow
7. fructose
8. starch
9. empty kcalorie
10. spend
11. nutrient
12. nutrition
13. protein
14. is not
15. physical activity
16. several
17. chromium
18. rare
19. ten
20. sugar, lowering
21. obese
22. hunger
23. control, sugar
24. obesity
25. do not
26. hardening, arteries
27. everyone
28. acid byproduct
29. starch
30. granola
31. cariogenicity
32. 20
33. may
34. the same
35. poor
36. poisonous

37. maybe
38. no
39. no
40. maybe
41. moderation

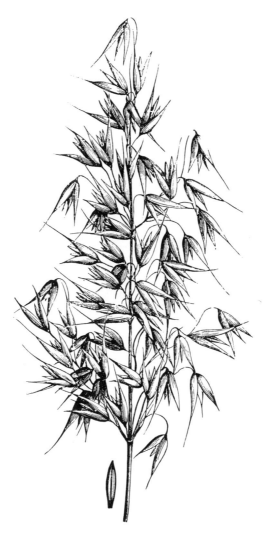

SELF TEST

1. Maintenance of the blood glucose level in the body:
    a. depends on replenishing from liver glycogen
        stores when too low.
    b. depends on siphoning off excess into storage when
        too high.
    c. can be made more stable by eating of complex
        carbohydrate foods.
    d. helps prevent symptoms of hypoglycemia such as
        dizziness and weakness.
    e. all of the above

2. The cells of your brain and nervous system normally depend
    on _____ for energy.
    a. what you eat
    b. glucose
    c. stored fat
    d. glucagon

3. The first organ to respond to raised blood glucose is:
    a. the liver.
    b. the pancreas.
    c. the brain.
    d. the stomach.

4. If you haven't eaten for a while, and your brain and other
    body cells need glucose, it will be supplied from
    _____ from the liver.
    a. insulin
    b. stored fat
    c. glucose
    d. glucagon
    e. protein

5. A hormone secreted by the pancreas to raise blood glucose
    is:
    a. glucose.
    b. glucagon.
    c. insulin.
    d. pancreatic juice.

6. Cells that secrete insulin are called _____ cells.
    a. alpha   c. gamma
    b. beta   d. theta

7. The chemical formula for glucose is:
    a. $C_{12}H_6O_{12}$
    b. $C_6H_{12}O_6$
    c. $C_6H_6O_{12}$

8. The normal blood glucose concentration range is _____
    mg/100ml.
    a. 40-60
    b. 60-80
    c. 80-120
    d. 120-160

9. Too much glucose in the blood is called:
    a. normoglycemia.
    b. hyperglycemia.
    c. hypoglycemia.

10. Too little glucose in the blood is called:
    a. normoglycemia.
    b. hyperglycemia.
    c. hypoglycemia.

11. A condensation reaction can:
    a. join two monosaccharides to form a disaccharide.
    b. take apart a disaccharide to produce two.
        monosaccharides.
    c. form a molecule of water.
    d. a and c
    e. b and c

12.   A hydrolysis reaction can:
      a.   join two monosaccharides to form a disaccharide.
      b.   take apart a disaccharide to produce two
      monsaccharides.
      c.   form a molecule of water.
      d.   a and c
      e.   b and c

13.   The facilitators of condensation and hydrolysis reactions
      are: _____
      a.   molecules of hot water.
      b.   enzymes.
      c.   hormones.
      d.   nutrients.
      14 -16. Use the following letters to answer questions 14,
      15 and 16:
            a.   one   b.   two   c.   three   d.   four   e.   none

14.   A carbon atom can form _____ (bond/bonds).

15.   An oxygen atom can form _____ (bond/bonds).

16.   A hydrogen atom forms _____ (bond/bonds).

17.   Which of the following is a complex carbohydrate?
      a.   glucose
      b.   starch
      c.   lactose
      d.   dextrose

18.   Sucrose is made up of:
      a.   two molecules of glucose.
      b.   glucose and fructose.
      c.   glucose and galacose.
      d.   two molecules of fructose.

19.   Monosaccharides include all of the following except:
      a.   glucose.
      b.   sucrose.
      c.   galactose.
      d.   fructose.

20.   Disaccharides include all of the following except:
      a.   sucrose.
      b.   lactose.
      c.   maltose.
      d.   fructose.

21. Carbohydrates are made of long branched chains of:
    a. double bonds.
    b. glycerol units.
    c. saccharide units.
    d. peptide linkages.

22. If hundreds of glucose units are strung together we say the resulting compound is a:
    a. polysaccharide.
    b. disaccharide.
    c. glyceride.
    d. glucoride.

23. The main use of carbohydrates by the body is:
    a. to provide energy.
    b. to insulate the body.
    c. to fuel the brain.

24. Lactose intolerance is caused by:
    a. an allergy to milk.
    b. drinking too much milk.
    c. excessive synthesis of lactase.
    d. inadequate synthesis of lactase.

25. Sugar causes tooth decay by:
    a. providing food for bacteria.
    b. adhering to teeth, causing enamel disintegration.
    c. combining with saliva to produce acid.

26. Which of the following compounds is a component of dietary fiber?
    a. lignin
    b. pectin
    c. cellulose
    d. hemicellulose
    e. all of the above

27. A suggested daily intake of crude fiber is about:
    a. 4-7 grams.
    b. 25 grams.
    c. 100 grams.
    d. none of the above.

28. One gram of carbohydrate supplies _____ kcalories.
    a. 2
    b. 4
    c. 6
    d. 9

Use the answers below for 29-33: (can use answer more than once).
    a. 5   b. 10   c. 12   d. 15   e. 20

29. One milk exchange provides _____ g of carbohydrate.

30. One vegetable exchange provides _____ g of carbohydrate.

31. One fruit exchange provides _____ g of carbohydrate.

32. One bread exchange provides _____ g of carbohydrate.

33. One teaspoon of molasses provides _____ g of carbohydrate.

34. Food fiber_____(is/is not) kcalorie-free.
    a. is   b. is not

35. The substance in food called _____ could cause losses of zinc, iron, calcium, copper, and magnesium.
    a. ascorbic acid
    b. phytic acid
    c. arachidonic acid
    d. linoleic acid

36. Which of the substances named is not an alternative sweetener?
    a. mannitol
    b. sorbitol
    c. xylitol
    d. aspartame

37. Which of the substances named is <u>not</u> an artificial sweetener?
    a. aspartame
    b. cyclamate
    c. saccharin
    d. sorbitol

38. White sugar, after digestion, yields a fifty-fifty mixture of glucose and _____ .
    a. fructose
    b. lactose
    c. polysaccharides
    d. maltose

39. In most of the world, when sugar consumption increases there is as much as a _____-fold increase in diabetes.
    a. hundred
    b. ten
    c. fifty
    d. three
    e. seven

40. Is sugar "bad" for you?
    a. yes
    b. no
    c. maybe

41. Is sugar "good for you?
    a. yes
    b. no
    c. maybe

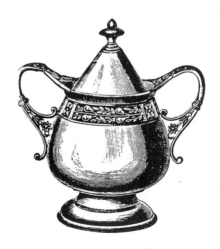

CHAPTER 2: SELF TEST ANSWERS

ANSWERS

1. e
2. b
3. b
4. c
5. b
6. b
7. b
8. c
9. b
10. c
11. d
12. b
13. b
14. d
15. c
16. a
17. b
18. b
19. b
20. d
21. c
22. a
23. a
24. d
25. a
26. e
27. a
28. b
29. c
30. a
31. b
32. d
33. a
34. b
35. b
36. d

CHAPTER 2: SELF TEST ANSWERS

37. d
38. a
39. b
40   c
41. b

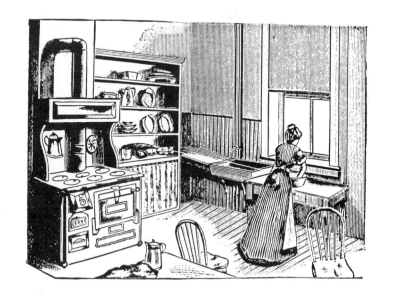

RECIPES YOU CAN TRY. . .

WHAT TO KNOW WHEN BUYING RICE

White Rice - Regular white rice has the outer coating of bran removed during milling. It comes in long, medium, or short grain forms. It is usually enriched with some of the vitamins which were lost during processing.

Unprocessed Brown Rice - Brown rice is the whole, unpolished form of rice. It has a nut-like flavor and is slightly chewy. It is highest in natural vitamins, minerals, and fiber.

"Converted" Rice (Uncle Ben's, is one trade name) - This is long-grain white rice which has been through a steam pressure process before milling which forces the B-vitamins into the grain. Then when the bran layer is removed the nutrients are not all lost. When cooked, the rice is very dry and fluffy.

"Instant," "Minute," or Quick-Cooking Rice - White rice is cooked to a mush and then extruded through special machinery to resemble rice kernels. The short cooking period merely rehydrates the rice pieces from their dehydrated form.

Important: Read the label on boxes of rice very carefully. The enrichment may be on the surface and can be lost by washing. Never rinse rice after cooking (see directions below). Bulk-packaged rice may have not been cleaned and may contain stones, twigs, grass and other matter.

How To Cook Brown Rice and White Rice

Bring two cups of water to a boil in a pan with a very tight-fitting cover. Add one teaspoon of salt and 1 cup of clean rice. Stir and immediately put cover on pan. Turn burner to lowest setting (warm on electric ranges, very low on gas). Set timer. White rice will be done in 20 minutes, brown in 45. If rice tends to burn, heat is too high. Try not to lift the lid during the cooking period until the very last. The rice can be "relaxed" by standing in covered pan an additional ten minutes after cooking and the grains will then easily separate.

RECIPES YOU CAN TRY. . .

RICE PUDDING

2 to 2-1/2 cups cooked brown rice   1/4 tsp cinnamon
1/3 cup raisins or dates   1 tbsp soft butter
1-1/3 cups milk   3 - 4 eggs
6 tbsp honey or brown sugar   1/2 tsp grated lemon rind
1/8 tsp salt   1 tsp lemon juice

Combine rice and raisins or dates in a greased 2-qt. baking
dish. Combine the remaining ingredients in a separate bowl or
blender container and beat or blend well. Pour this mixture
over the rice and stir together lightly with a fork. Bake the
pudding at 325° for about 1 hour or until pudding is set.
Test it by sticking a table knife in the center--it should come
out clean. Serves 6-8.

Did you know that rice makes a great, nutritious breakfast?
Stir in raisins, cinnamon, sugar, and milk for delicious hot
cereal.

Rice can be frozen and re-used at a later date. Leftover rice
can be tossed onto soups, salads, casseroles, or vegetable
dishes or blended into sauces and gravies.

RED BEANS AND RICE

1 (1-1b.) can kidney or red beans
Water
1 cup regular long-grain white rice
1-1/2 cups sliced onion
1 tsp. garlic salt
1 tsp salt
1 tsp chili powder

Drain kidney beans; reserve juice. Add water as needed to make
2-1/2 cups liquid. In a large skillet, combine kidney beans,
liquid, rice, onion, garlic salt, salt and chili powder. Stir.
Bring to a boil and cover. Simmer 20 minutes. Remove from heat.
Let stand, covered, until all liquid is absorbed, about 5
minutes. Makes 4 to 6 servings.

This could be cooked over a campfire or hot plate. You can
substitute black-eyed peas for kidney or red beans.

Variations:

Sprinkle with 1 cup shredded Cheddar cheese at end of 20 minutes
cooking time. Cover and let stand to melt cheese and absorb
liquid.

CHAPTER 3
The Lipids: Fats and Oils

YOU WILL LEARN...

1. The roles of fats and oils.

2. What a chemist sees when analyzing fats.

3. How fat is handled by the body.

4. The name and importance of the essential fatty acid.

5. What is different about processed fat.

6. What ketones are.

7. That triglycerides comprise 95% of body lipids and are named for their structure.

8. How cis to trans change occurs in fatty acids, and the health implications this might have.

9. How the phospholipids and sterols, making up 5% of body lipids, differ from the triglycerides.

10. What is good about cholesterol.

11. What helps the body to excrete cholesterol rather than deposit it abnormally.

12. What the Dietary Goals recommend regarding fat in the diet.

13.   Which exchange lists include fat.

14.   About a new, artificial fat.

HIGHLIGHT 3:   NUTRITION AND ATHEROSCLEROSIS

15.   What atherosclerosis is.

16.   What the risk factors implicated in heart disease are and which three are most important.

17.   Whether you can raise your HDL level and lower LDL and what this has to do with the risk of heart disease.

CHAPTER 3: THE LIPIDS: FATS AND OILS

THE LIPIDS: FATS AND OILS

1. About a _____ of the world's population is
    underfed, and at least a _____ of our population is
    overfed.

2. The lipids are a family of compounds that include both
    _____ and _____.

3. Fats and oils help keep you healthy by:
    a. Helping keep skin and hair normal,
    b. Insulating the body from temperature change,
    c. Protecting mammary glands, and
    d. Providing _____ for muscles and other tissues.

4. To go totally without an energy supply, even for a few
    minutes, would be to _____.

5. When liver glycogen is depleted, the body must receive new
    food or start degrading body _____ to continue
    making glucose.

6. The body's fat stores can provide _____ or even more
    of the body's ongoing energy need during food deprivation.

7. Fat cells are also called _____ cells.

8. One pound of body fat provides _____ kcalories.

9. Although fat provides energy in a fast, it cannot do so in
    the form of _____, so lean _____ _____
    is also broken down.

10. Half of the energy needs of the brain and nervous system
    can be met by _____ after a long period of glucose
    deprivation.

CHAPTER 3: THE LIPIDS: FATS AND OILS

FAT IN FOODS

11. Many compounds that give foods their _____ and _____ are found in fats and oils.

12. Vitamins A, D, _____, and _____ are fat soluble.

13. When the fat and water in a food separate, the other compounds in the food must go with either the _____ or the _____.

14. Besides flavor, aroma, and vitamins, _____ are also lost when fat is removed from food.

15. The single most effective step you can take to reduce the energy value of a food is to eat it without the _____.

The Chemist's view of Fats

16. Almost all (95 percent) of the lipids in the diet are _____.

17. The other two classes of dietary lipids are the _____ and the _____.

18. Cholesterol is a _____.

The Triglycerides

19. Triglycerides are named for their structure; they all have a "backbone" of _____ to which _____ fatty acids are attached.

20. A fatty acid is a chain of carbon atoms with hydrogens attached and with an _____ group (COOH) at one end.

21. When fatty acids are loaded with all the hydrogen atoms they can carry, they are called _____.

22. If some Hs were to be removed, the result would be an _____ or even _____ fat.

23. It is important to know that the structure determines the type of fat and how it is handled in the body. The three important classifications are: saturated, monounsaturated, and _____.

CHAPTER 3:   THE LIPIDS: FATS AND OILS

The Essential Fatty Acids

24. The term essential, when used in nutrition, means somthing that has to be supplied by the diet in food. _____ is an essential fatty acid.

25. Another important fatty acid, _____ acid, can be made from linoleic acid in the body when necessary.

26. Linolenic is often confused with linoleic. However, it--like arachidonic--can probably be made by the body if _____ acid is supplied.

27. The body's cells can convert one compound to another. In fact, triglycerides can be made from _____.

28. The dietary of essential fatty acids can be small, only _____ of corn oil per day would be sufficient.

29. It is difficult sometimes to prove the relationship between symptoms and _____.

The Prostaglandins

30. Hormone-like compounds produced in the body from the essential fatty acids are called _____.

31. Rather than having names, they are designated by letters and _____.

Processed Fat

32. The degree of unsaturation of a fat can be determined chemically by obtaining an "_____ number."

33. The more polyunsaturated a product is, the more it loses in keeping _____.

34. A chemical process by which hydrogen atoms are added to unsaturated or polyunsaturated fats is called: _____.

35. In partially hydrogenated or heated polyunsaturated fats, a change in the chemical structure occurs changing the configuration from cis (the same side) to _____ (the opposite side).

36. The cis-trans shift may make us prone to developing some types of _____.

CHAPTER 3: THE LIPIDS: FATS AND OILS

How the Body Handles Fat

37. Water-fearing substances are hydrophobic or _____.

38. Water-loving substances are _____.

39. _____ _____ are needed to prepare the fat for digestion.

40. When fat is broken up, dispersed, and stabilized in a watery solution it is _____. Before entry into the intestinal cells, it forms particles known as _____.

41. The emulsifying compound manufactured by the liver is called _____. It stored in the _____.

42. When the enzymes dismantle the triglycerides for digestion, the units usable by the body are monoglycerides, _____, and fatty acids--which pass into the cells of the intestinal wall.

43. When the larger lipids are prepared for transport throughout the body, they are wrapped in protein and called _____.

The Phospholipids

44. The phospholipids and _____ comprise only _____ percent of the lipids in the diet.

45. The best known of the phospholipids are the _____.

46. A phospholipid is similar to a _____ but has choline or another substance in place of one of the fatty acids.

47. The lecithin you eat does _____ reach the body tissues intact. In fact the lecithin you need for building cell membranes is made from scratch by the _____.

48. Another function of lecithin is to act as an _____.

CHAPTER 3: THE LIPIDS: FATS AND OILS

THE STEROLS: CHOLESTEROL

49. Molecules similar to cholesterol include the bile acids, adrenocortical hormones, _____ hormones, and vitamin _____.

50. Cholesterol _____ (is/is not) an essential nutrient.

51. Cholesterol can be made from either _____ or fat.

52. The cholesterol that leaves the liver:
    a. May be made into bile,
    b. May be deposited in body tissues,
    c. May accumulate in the _____.

How Cholesterol is Excreted

53. (See diagram on the recycling of cholesterol and bile.) Some cholesterol can become part of the _____ salts that help emulsify _____.

54. While in the intestine, bile salts can be trapped by certain kinds of _____ _____, thereby reducing the total amount of cholesterol that is absorbed.

How Cholesterol is Deposited in the Body

55. Some cholesterol leaves the liver in packages for use by the body tissues. These packages are the _____.

56. More than _____ of all the body's cholesterol is located in the cells.

57. To pass into the cells, lipids must first cross the _____ walls.

The Fats in Foods

58. The Dietary Goals, translated into the Dietary Guidelines, recommend avoiding excess fat, saturated fat, and _____.

59. The consumption of total fat in the diet today is _____ (higher/lower) than it was in 1972.

60. People probably do eat about _____ to _____ % of their kcalories as fat.

61. _____ of the six lists in the exchange system include
     foods containing fat.

62. There are nine kcalories per gram of fat, and in a teaspoon
     there are _____ grams of fat, or 45 calories.

63. Meat, which is thought of as a protein food, actually often
     contains more _____ energy than _____ energy.

64. The weight of meat portions in the exchange system is only
     _____ ounce. (do not confuse this with "serving size"
     when using the Four Food Group System.)

     One important classification of fats is determining whether
     they are saturated or unsaturated (or polyunsaturated).
     Your first clue is this: products containing saturated
     fats tend to be solid at room temperature, unsaturated tend
     to be liquid.

65. Lard, butter, bacon or ham fat, beef fat or meat "marbling"
     are examples of _____ fat.

66. Most vegetable oils are mono or polyunsaturated. Olive oil
     is an example of a _____ fat.

67. Coconut oil is a _____ fat.

68. High blood pressure is related to a high _____
     (fat/sodium) intake.

ARTIFICIAL FAT: SUCROSE POLYESTER

69. A synthetic combination of sucrose and fatty acids that
     looks, feels, and tastes like food fat but is indigestible
     is _____ _____.

70. SPE is _____ (digestible/indigestible), and so
     far appears to be _____ (safe/unsafe).

71. It may be helpful in solving two of our major health
     problems, _____ and _____ blood,
     cholesterol.

SUMMING UP

(refer to textbook for summary)

ANSWERS

1. third, third
2. fats, oils
3. energy
4. die
5. protein
6. 2/3
7. adipose
8. 3,500
9. glucose, body tissue
10. ketones
11. flavor, aroma
12. E,K
13. fat, water
14. kcalories
15. fat
16. triglycerides
17. phospholipids, sterols
18. sterol
19. glycerol, three
20. acid
21. saturated
22. unsaturated, polyunsaturated
23. polyunsaturated
24. linoleic acid
25. arachidonic
26. linoleic
27. glucose
28. one teaspoon
29. nutrients
30. prostaglandins
31. numbers
32. iodine
33. quality
34. hydrogenation
35. trans
36. cancer
37. lipophilic
38. hydrophilic
39. Bile acids
40. emulsified, micelles
41. bile, gallbladder
42. glycerol
43. lipoproteins
44. sterols
45. lecithins

46.   triglyceride
47.   not, liver
48.   emulsifying agent
49.   sex, D
50.   is not
51.   carbohydrate
52.   arteries
53.   bile, fat
54.   dietary fiber
55.   lipoproteins
56.   nine-tenths
57.   artery
58.   cholesterol
59.   lower
60.   40 - 50
61.   Three
62.   five
63.   fat, protein
64.   one
65.   saturated
66.   mono-unsaturated
67.   saturated
68.   sodium
69.   sucrose polyester
70.   indigestible, safe
71.   obesity, high

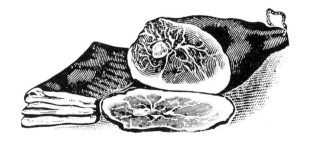

HIGHLIGHT 3:   NUTRITION AND ATHEROSCLEROSIS

1. More than _____ of the people who die in the United States each year die of heart and blood vessel disease.

2. The underlying condition that contributes to most of these deaths is _____.

3. Artery disease often begins with a condition called _____ of the arteries.

4. In atherosclerosis, soft mounds of _____ accumulate along the inner walls of the arteries. They are called _____.

5. When the arteries cannot expand normally, the blood pressure _____.

6. If the artery weakens and balloons out, it is called an _____ which can burst, causing death.

7. Plaques can also cause the clotting _____ to begin, which could lead to a heart _____ or _____.

8. Atherosclerosis begins _____. Most individuals have well developed plaques by the time they are _____.

9. The abbreviation "CHD" means _____ _____ _____.

10. The abbreviationn "CVD" Means _____ _____ _____.

11. Factors known to be related to a disease but not known to be causal are called _____ _____.

12. Factors linked to atherosclerosis include being male, heredity, high blood pressure, lack of exercise, obesity. stress, high blood fats, nutrient excesses or deficiencies, personality traits, and _____.

13. The three major risk factors seem to be smoking, high blood cholesterol, and _____ blood pressure.

14. "High blood cholesterol" is considered to be any value over _____ mg/100 ml.

15. The opposite of a "retrospective" study is a "_____"study.

16. "Type A" personalities are _____ (more/less) likely to develop heart disease.

Intervention studies

17. Statistics show that between the late 1960s and the late 1970s, deaths from CVD _____.

How to Lower Serum Cholesterol

18. In interpreting statistics, note that there is an important difference between _____ cholesterol and _____ cholesterol.

19. Dietary fat and cholesterol are the "fat on the _____."

20. Serum triglycerides and cholesterol are the "fat in the _____."

21. Dietary cholesterol_____ (does/does not) raise cholesterol in the blood very much.

22. Saturated fat (on the plate) raises _____ (in the blood).

23. High _____ cholesterol is an indicator of risk for CVD, and the main food factor associated with it is a high _____ fat intake.

24. The two vehicles that carry cholesterol in the blood are the low-density lipoproteins (LDL) and the _____ -density ones (HDL). The LDL seem to "feed" the plaques and we want to lower this fraction as much as possible. The HDL are the "good guys" and may inhibit plaque formation.

25. Influential factors in diet regarding cholesterol are:
    a. Saturated fat--which_____ serum cholesterol (LDL).
    b. Monounsaturated and polyunsaturated fat--which _____ it.
    c. Cholesterol itself--which raises if slightly, depending on the amount eaten and on the body's ability to compensate by making _____.

26. Dietary fiber may also confer _____.

27. Persons on _____ _____ diets excrete more bile acids, sterols, and fat than persons on low-fiber diets.

28. Soluble fibers such as _____ and guar gum, lower the cholesterol more than the insoluble fibers such as _____ and lignin. Therefore, rolled oats, apples, oranges, and other fruits are more favorable than _____ bran.

29. A diet less controversial than the Pritikin diet, and developed by the American Heart Association, is the _____ Diet, which regulates fat and cholesterol at slightly lower levels than the average.

30. How to Raise HDL
    a. Stop smoking   d. Eat more fish than meat
    b. Be female   e. Increase certain fibers in diet
    c. Lose weight   but above all,
                            f. _____.

31. CVD deaths are _____ while others are on the _____.

32. Two possible food-borne causes of atherosclerosis currently under investigation involve an enzyme in cow's milk and the possibility that oxidation products of _____ and vitamin D in processed foods.
    If at all possible, refer to some of the resources given so that you will have a chance to read a research paper for yourself and understand the difficulty of making absolute statements.

ANSWERS

1. half
2. atherosclerosis
3. hardening
4. lipids, plaques
5. rises
6. aneurysm
7. reaction, attack, stroke
8. early, thirty
9. coronary heart disease
10. cardio vascular disease
11. risk factors
12. smoking
13. high
14. 220
15. prospective
16. more
17. decreased
18. dietary, serum
19. plate
20. blood
21. does not
22. cholesterol
23. serum, saturated
24. high
25. a. raises
    b. lowers
    c. less
26. benefits
27. high fiber
28. pectin, cellulose, wheat
29. Prudent
30. exercise
31. falling, rise
32. cholesterol

CHAPTER 3: THE LIPIDS: FATS AND OILS

SELF TEST

1. You can't be too thin.
    a. true
    b. false

2. The lipids:
    a. include fats but not oils.
    b. include oils but not fats.
    c. include both fats and oils.

3. To go totally without an energy supply, even for a few minutes, would be:
    a. an easy way to keep from getting fat.
    b. restful to our vital organs.
    c. to die.
    d. hard for a person with good appetite.

4. Without a food supply, energy for the brain is produced:
    a. first from glycogen, next from body protein.
    b. by destroying fat cells.
    c. both of the above.
    d. neither of the above

5. A pound of body fat supplies:
    a. 2,000 kcal.
    b. 500 kcal.
    c. 3,000 kcal.
    d. 3,500 kcal.
    e. none of the above

6. A condensation product of fat metabolism, produced when carbohydrate is not available is called:
    a. atrophy
    b. ketones
    c. lipids

7. Body fat does all <u>except</u>:
    a. maintain health of skin and hair.
    b. protect body organs from temperature extremes.
    c. provide a continuous fuel supply.
    d. provide glucose for the brain and nerves.
    e. protect organs from shock.

8. When fat is removed from a food:
    a. kcalories are lost.
    b. vitamins are lost.
    c. flavor is lost.
    d. all of the above
    e. none of the above

9. Triglycerides make up _____ of the lipids in the
    diet.
    a. 50%.
    b. 75%.
    c. 95%.
    d. 100%.
    e. none of the above

10. All glycerol molecules are alike, but the fatty acids may
     vary in two ways:
     a. length and degree of saturation.
     b. saturation and unsaturation.
     c. glycerol molecules and fatty acids.

11. A polyunsaturated fat contains triglycerides in which the
     fatty acids may be:
     a. long, medium or short.
     b. saturated or unsaturated.
     c. glycerol molecules or chains.
     d. a and b

12. If the fatty acids attached to the glycerol backbones of
     triglycerides are fully loaded with hydrogen atoms, we say
     the fat is
     a. unsaturated.
     b. saturated.
     c. polyunsaturated.

13. The essential fatty acid/s (is/are):
     a. linoleic.
     b. linolenic.
     c. arachadonic.
     d. bucolic.
     e. a,b,and c.

14. There is a consistent relationship between symptoms and
    nutrients.
    a. true
    b. false

15. Further, there is always a link between foods and symptoms.
    a. true
    b. false

16. Hormone-like compounds produced in the body from the
    essential fatty acids are called:
    a. prostaglandins.
    b. PUFA.
    c. triglycerides.
    d. trans-fatty acids.

17. Unusual molecules arise when unsaturated fats are partially
    hydrogenated. These molecules may create problems in our
    cells and tissues because they are not made by the body's
    cells and are rare in foods. They are called:
    a. trans-fatty acids.
    b. cis-fatty acids.
    c. non-essential fatty acids.
    d. hydrogenated fatty acids.
    e. sucrose polyester.

18. Bile acids needed to prepare fats for digestion are made
    largely from:
    a. cholesterol.
    b. lipids.
    c. linoleic acid.
    d. stearic acid.

19. When the products of lipid digestion are released for
    transport throughout the body, some of the larger ones are
    packaged in protein for this purpose. The packages are
    called:
    a. carboxyl units.
    b. lipidemia molecules.
    c. lipoproteins.
    d. protein-fat packages.

20. Five percent of the lipids in the diet are comprised of:
    a.   phospholipids.
    b.   sterols.
    c.   triglycerides.
    d.   a and b
    e.   cholesterol.

21. One of the phospholipids needed for building cell membranes is:
    a.   cholesterol.
    b.   lecithin.
    c.   glycerol.
    d.   a sterol.

22. Cholesterol can be made in the liver from either:
    a.   carbohydrate or fat.
    b.   saturated or unsaturated fats.
    c.   eggs or bacon.
    d.   none of the above.

23. Which of the following is not true true about cholesterol:

    a.   When it leaves the liver it may be deposited in
         body tissues.
    b.   When it leaves the liver it may be excreted in
         the feces.
    c.   It may wind up accumulating in arteries and
         causing artery disease.
    d.   It may be made into bile, move into the intestine,
         and some may then be excreted in the feces.

24. More than five-tenths of all the body's cholesterol is
    located:
    a.   in the arteries.
    b.   in the cells.
    c.   in the liver.
    d.   in the brain.

25. An artificial fat made of sugar and fatty acids which adds
    no calories and looks, feels, and tastes like food fat is
    called:
    a.   diet-fat.
    b.   thin and slim.
    c.   sucrose polyester.
    d.   SPE oil.

26. A fatty acid that has one double bond is:
    a. saturated.
    b. monounsaturated.
    c. polyunsaturated.
    d. hydrogenated.

27. A fatty acid with two or more double bonds is described as:
    a. saturated.
    b. monounsaturated.
    c. polyunsaturated.
    d. hydrogenated.

28. A component of food that may lower serum cholesterol is:
    a. pectin.
    b. bran.
    c. wheat germ.
    d. seeds.

29. The following are thought to help remove cholesterol from the body:
    a. HDL.
    b. LDL.
    c. VLDL.
    d. chylomicrons.

30. Cholesterol is not :
    a. found in food.
    b. synthesized in the body.
    c. found in brain tissue.
    d. the precursor of the sex hormones.
    e. a fatty acid.

31. Of the six lists in the exchange system, _____ contain quite a bit of fat.
    a. two.
    b. three.
    c. four.
    d. five.

32. Fat contains _____ kcalories per gram and there are five grams per teaspoon.
    a. three.
    b. four.
    c. seven.
    d. nine.
    e. twelve.

HIGHLIGHT 3:   NUTRITION AND ATHEROSCLEROSIS

33. The three factors which are the major predictors of risk
     for heart disease are all <u>but:</u>
     a. smoking.
     b. high serum cholesterol.
     c. high blood pressure.
     d. stress.

34. High blood cholesterol is any value over _____
     mg/100ml.
     a. 120.
     b. 200.
     c. 220.
     d. 350.
     e. 500.

35. High serum cholesterol and high dietary cholesterol are
     both indicators of probable heart disease.
     a. true
     b. false

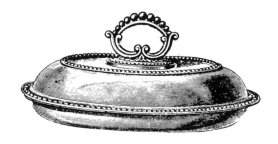

ANSWERS

1. b
2. c
3. c
4. a
5. d
6. b
7. d
8. d
9. c
10. a
11. d
12. b
13. e
14. b
15. b
16. a
17. a
18. a
19. c
20. d
21. b
22. a
23. a
24. b
25. c
26. b
27. c
28. a
29. a
30. e
31. b
32. d
33. d
34. c
35. b

MAKING CHOICES

The controversy regarding butter vs. margarine, or which oil to use in the kitchen, is a complicated one. A very informative analysis of how to apply scientific findings to everyday buying and cooking is contained in The Supermarket Handbook.* Because of the hydrogenation of fat in most margarines as well as the many additives allowed, a sparse use of butter itself may be a better choice. There are, in addition, alternative spreads for bread that may be considered such as ricotta cheese, tahina (sesame butter), mashed avocado or cottage cheese moistened with skim milk.

Some cooks favor olive oil since it is cold-pressed and totally unrefined with no additives. It can be purchased by the gallon at reasonable cost at wholesale grocery outlets and can be used for everything except frying. Peanut oil, soybean oil, and sunflower oil are excellent all-purpose oils. Safflower and corn oils are good choices if you can find them without preservatives.

The following recipe is a way to stretch butter, increase polysaturates, and avoid hydrogenation and additives. Since it is easy to spread less is used and thus calories reduced.

BUTTER SPREAD

In a blender container put the following ingredients:
    2 sticks softened butter (not melted)
    1 cup salad oil (see above for suggestions)
    2 tbsp water, 2 tbsp dried skim milk
    1/2 tsp lecithin granules (available at health food stores)

Blend until creamy and pour into small containers. Refrigerate except when being used.

(Hint: Wash your blender immediately. Oil attacks rubber parts if left on and wears them out faster.)

RECIPES YOU CAN TRY...

ONE-APPLE PIE

This pie is made from only one apple and makes two generous servings. Even beginners and children over the age of 8 can have good luck with this.

First make pastry: In a bowl combine
1/3 cup unsifted regular flour
1 tsp sugar, 2 tbsp butter

Rub with fingers until evenly mixed. With a fork, stir in 1 tbsp milk until dough holds together. Press into a ball and cut in half. Roll out one portion on a floured board until large enough to fit a 4 or 5 inch pie pan, with some pastry extending beyond rim.

Peel and core 1 medium-large Golden Delicious or Newtown Pippin apple and slice fruit. Mix with 1 to 2 tbsp sugar and 1/4 tsp cinnamon. Pile fruit into pastry-lined pan. Roll out remaining pastry until large enough to cover apples. Fold pastry edges together to seal in fruit, then crimp rim. Prick top and bake pie on lowest rack in a 375 degree oven for 45 minutes or until crust is well browned and pie bubbles.

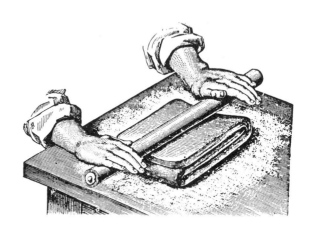

*Goldbeck, N & D. The Supermarket Handbook. New York: The New American Library, 1976.

CHAPTER 4

Protein: Amino Acids

YOU WILL LEARN

1. How the extraordinary structure of proteins makes them the most versatile of the energy nutrients.

2. What a chemist sees when viewing protein.

3. Amino acid structures, and how condensation reactions connect them.

4. How amino acids are sequenced into proteins.

5. How folding and tangling of the chains makes giant protein molecules.

6. How protein is denatured.

7. About the complexity and variety of proteins used in the body.

8. How enzymes work and what they are made of.

9. To understand the "protein circle."

10. How enzymes alter compounds.

11. How protein quality is measured, and what the "reference protein" is.

12. About the other roles of protein.

13. How proteins are transported.

14. About protein-kcalorie malnutrition: kwashiorkor, marasmus, and alcoholism.

CHAPTER 4:   PROTEIN AND AMINO ACIDS

15. About recommended protein intakes, and nitrogen balance.

16. The <u>Dietary Goals</u> for protein.

17. Whether we can get too much protein.

18. What foods contain protein.

HIGHLIGHT 4:   NUTRITION AND THE BRAIN

19. The effect of certain foods on the brain

20. How to use nutrition knowledge to enhance brain function
     and well being.

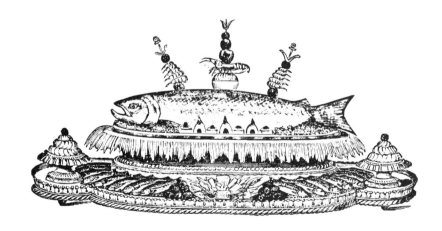

CHAPTER 4:   PROTEIN AND AMINO ACIDS

PROTEIN

1. The most important of all the known organic substances in living matter is _____.

2. One thing that protein does <u>not</u> do for you is make you _____.

3. Protein is composed of carbon, hydrogen, _____, and _____ atoms. Some amino acids also contain _____ atoms.

4. There are _____ different common amino acids that link together to form proteins. They connect by means of a _____ _____. The bond forming as the two amino acids condense is called a _____ bond.

5. Two amino acids bonded together with a peptide bond are called a _____. Three are a _____ and many are a_____.

6. When a protein's shape changes due to heat, acid, or other conditions, the protein is said to be _____, this change is irreversible past a certain point.

ENZYMES: A FUNCTION OF PROTEIN

7. A word ending in "ase" such as protease, lipase, or lactase, designates an _____ which hydrolyzes protein, lipids, lactose, etc.

8. A _____ is a compound that facilitates chemical reactions itself being destroyed in the process.

9. An _____ is a protein catalyst.

10.   The genetic code of the _____ determines protein
       sequences.

11.   Review the protein story: All enzymes are proteins, all
       proteins are made of amino acids. Amino acids have to be
       put together to make protein. _____ put together
       the amino acids.

A Closer Look at Enzyme Action

(If your instructor stresses learning the biochemical pathway of
these compounds, review in text.)

12.   The role of protein is to supply the amino acids from which
       the body can make its own _____.

PROTEIN QUALITY

13.   There are _____ essential amino acids for adults, plus
       _____ for infants.

14.   The first important characteristic of dietary protein is
       that it should supply at least the _____ essential
       amino acids and enough _____ for the synthesis of
       the others.

15.   Complete protein_____ (is/is not) the same as
       high-quality protein.

16.   The limiting amino acid in a protein is the one found in
       the _____ supply relative to the amount needed for
       protein synthesis in the body.

17.   The "reference protein," assigned a biological value of
       100, is _____ protein.

18.   Comparing a test protein's amino acid composition with that
       of a reference protein results in a _____ _____.

19.   Since protein varies in digestibility, chemical scoring
       does not always reflect accurately the way the body will
       use _____.

CHAPTER 4: PROTEIN AND AMINO ACIDS

20. "Predigested" protein is_____ (more/less) absorbable than whole protein.

21. A better test for protein usability is _____ _____.

22. Still another indication of protein usability, involving feeding young animals, is called _____ _____ ratio, or PER.

23. Taking gelatin _____ (helps/doesn't help) cracked nails or brittle hair.

24. Which comes first in the body, protein needs or energy needs? _____.

25. Carbohydrate and fat have a protein-_____ action.

OTHER ROLES OF PROTEIN

26. When protein performs other important roles, other _____ maybe needed to assist it in ways that the student will understand better in subsequent chapters.

Fluid balances

27. Proteins help <u>maintain</u> the water _____.

28. The space in the blood vessels is the _____ space.

29. The space between the cells is the _____ or space.

30. The space inside the cells is the _____ space.

31. Water molecules stay with or near the _____ because proteins are _____.

32. The accumulation of fluid in the interstitial spaces is called _____.

33. You _____ (can/cannot) normally cause edema by drinking too much water.

34. The body maintains its own _____.

35. Taking diuretics _____ (does/does not) help to control body fat.

36.   Proteins help to maintain acid- _____ balance.

37.   The ability to regulate the acidity of the medium is known as the _____ action of proteins.

Antibodies and Hormones

38.   The antibodies are giant _____ molecules circulating in the blood defending us against viruses, bacteria, and other "foreign agents."

39.   Many hormones are made of amino _____ , such as the _____ hormone and _____.

Transport Proteins

40.   Some proteins specialize in moving _____ and other molecules in and out of cells.

41.   Permeases, vectorial enzymes, and transferases are other names for _____-associated proteins.

42.   Almost every water-soluble nutrient seems to have its own _____ system in cell membranes. Lipids, however, can cross without the help of _____.

43.   However, only the smaller lipids--monoglycerides, glycerol, and fatty acids--travel freely without carriers. The larger ones can travel in water only because of their _____ coats, and are called _____.

44.   The mineral iron illustrates how important _____ are in handling specific nutrients.

45.   At least one _____ is similarly involved in the body's handling of calcium.

46. The proteins involved in the intricate handling of iron all have special names:
    a.   The protein in the intestinal-wall cells is
    _____.
    b.   The carrier protein is _____.
    c.   The storage protein is _____ again.
    d.   The red-blood cell protein is _____.
    e.   The muscle-cell protein is _____.

CHAPTER 4: PROTEIN AND AMINO ACIDS

Blood Clotting

47. The stringy, insoluble mass of fibers that plugs the cut when we are wounded is called _____. Again, protein is involved along with helper nutrients such as Vitamin K.

Connective Tissue

48. Proteins help make scar _____, bones, and _____.

49. The protein material of which scars, tendons, ligaments, and the foundations of bones and teeth are made is called _____. Vitamin C and other minerals are the helper nutrients in this process.

Visual Pigments

50. The protein _____ makes up the molecules of the light-sensitive pigments in the cells of the retina.

PROTEIN DEFICIENCY

51. The world's most serious malnutrition problem is _____ - _____ deficiency.

52. The classic protein deficiency disease is _____ and the kcalorie deficiency disease is _____.

Kwashiorkor

53. Kwashiorkor occurs in wealthy, as well as _____, countries on every continent. Lack of the mineral _____ may also be involved.

54. In protein deficiency, the first body proteins to be lost are the _____ and _____ pigments.

55. Antibodies may be sacrificed to protect the heart, _____ and brain tissue.

56. Malnutrition and _____ are a deadly combination.

Marasmus

57. Marasmus is more than just a shortage of protein, it is a deficiency in _____ and most other nutrients.

58. Another aspect is _____, and there are multiple problems from the effects of nutritional, emotional and intellectual deprivation.

59. PCM especially affects vulnerable groups in the community such as pregnant and lactating women, _____ infants, just-weaned children, and children in periods of rapid growth.

Adult PCM

60. Most people don't think of alcoholics as having the same symptoms as one suffering from _____.

61. Adult kwashiorkor and marasmus also occur in hospital patients whose diets have been _____.

62. Hospital malnutrition occurs in up to _____ of hospital patients.

RECOMMENDED PROTEIN INTAKES

63. Proteins are needed for growth and _____ of all body tissues as well as for repair.

64. You even lose protein when you take a _____, or cut your fingernails or hair.

65. It is said that a person's skin is replaced totally every _____ years.

66. The quantity of protein that you need depends on the amount of _____ _____ in your body. (Note: it has virtually nothing to do with how active you are.)

67. Exactly how much protein is needed is determined by laboratory scientists who perform _____ balance studies.

68. Nitrogen balance is a measure of the nitrogen _____ (N in) as compared with the amount of nitrogen excreted (N out).

CHAPTER 4: PROTEIN AND AMINO ACIDS

69. Protein is estimated from the weight of the nitrogen multiplied by _____.

70. A person can be in nitrogen equilibrium, positive nitrogen balance(-where there is more coming in than going out-)or negative nitrogen balance (where there is more going out then _____ _____).

71. A healthy adult is probably in nitrogen _____.

72. Growing children and pregnant women are in _____ nitrogen balance.

73. People who are sick are often in _____ nitrogen balance, except those people with diseased kidneys.

The Dietary Goal for Protein

74. Protein intake has been relatively constant in U.S. diets and should remain at about _____ % of the kcalories in your diet.

75. Dietary goals for the three energy nutrients are:
    a. Protein, _____ of kcalories with a range of 10-15 percent.
    b. Carbohydrate, _____ of kcalories (or more).
    c. Fat, _____ of kcalories (or less).

(In calculating your percentage of kcalories from these energy nutrients remember that carbohydrate and protein both have 4 kcalories per gram; fat, 9. See text for calculations necessary.

The RDA for Protein

76. A generous protein allowance for a healthy adult is _____ grams of high-quality protein per kilogram of ideal body weight. (See text for calculation procedure.)

77. The RDA Committee assumes that the protein eaten will be of high quality (PER equal to that of _____ or above,) that it will be consumed with adequate kcalories from carbohydrate and _____, and that other nutrients will be adequate.

The Canadian and FAO/WHO Recommendations

78. The Canadian recommendation is _____ to the RDA.

79.   The protein recommendation of the world health agencies
      is_____g/kg.

80.   Generous intakes of protein in poorer countries would be a
      _____.

The Upper Limit

81.   It _____ (is/is not) possible to consume too much
      protein.

82.   The livers and kidneys of animals fed too much protein grow
      too _____ (hypertrophy).

83.   High protein diets promote calcium _____.

84.   The higher a person's intake of protein, the more likely
      that other important nutrients will be _____ out.

PROTEIN IN FOODS

85.   Using the exchange system, the two lists that provide good
      protein in abundance are the _____ and _____ list.

86.   The principles of wise diet planning are adequacy, balance,
      variety and _____.

SUMMING UP

Review summary in text.

Check with your instructor about whether you should memorize the
      names of the essential amino acids.

T _____   P _____
V _____   M _____

T _____
I _____
L _____
L _____

ANSWERS

1. protein
2. thin
3. oxygen, nitrogen, sulfur
4. 22, condensation reaction, dipeptide
5. dipeptide, tripeptide, polypeptide
6. denatured
7. enzyme
8. catalyst
9. enzyme
10. DNA
11. Enzymes
12. proteins
13. 8, histidine
14. 8, nitrogen
15. is not
16. shortest
17. egg
18. chemical score
19. protein
20. less
21. biological value
22. net protein, ratio
23. doesn't help
24. energy needs
25. sparing
26. nutrients
27. balance
28. intravascular
29. intercellular, interstitial
30. intracellular
31. proteins
    hydrophilic
32. edema
33. cannot
34. health
35. does not
36. base
37. buffering
38. protein
39. acids, thyroid, insulin
40. nutrients
41. membrane
42. transport, pumps
43. protein, lipoproteins
44. proteins
45. protein
46. a. ferritin

       b.   transferrin
       c.   ferritin
       d.   hemoglobin
       e.   myoglobin
47. fibrin
48. tissue, teeth
49. collagen
50. opsin
51. protein, Kcalorie
52. kwashiorkor, marasmus
53. poor, zinc
54. hair, skin
55. lungs
56. infection
57. kcalories
58. neglect
59. nursing
60. kwashiorkor
61. inadequate
62. 50%
63. maintenance
64. bath
65. seven
66. lean tissue
67. nitrogen
68. consumed
69. 6.25
70. coming in
71. equilibrium
72. positive
73. negative
74. 12
75. a.   12%
    b.   58%
    c.   30%
76. .8
77. casein, fat
78. similar
79. .75
80. luxury
81. is
82. large
83. excretion
84. crowded
85. milk, meat
86. moderation
    tryptophan, valine, threonine, isoleucine,
    lysine, leucine, phenylalanine, methionine

HIGHLIGHT 4:   NUTRITION AND THE BRAIN

1. Food _____ (does/does not) affect mood, behavior, and wakefulness.

2. The _____ selectively removes toxins, drugs, and excess quantities of nutrients.

3. The blood contents arriving at the brain have already been _____ adjusted and cleansed.

4. In addition, there is a _____-brain barrier.

5. If there is a _____ of an essential nutrient, the brain's supply falls _____.

6. Exceptions to the rule that substances in the brain don't reflect blood concentrations are the _____.

7. Nutrition is linked to brain activity in some _____ ways.

8. The gap between nerve cells, or between nerve and muscle cells, is called a _____.

9. A neurotransmitter can either stimulate or _____ the post-synaptic neuron.

10. Among the diet-responsive neurotransmitters are seroton in, acetylcholine, and _____.

11. A lack of _____ flowing into the brain can cause wakefulness, sensitivity to pain, and possible _____.

12. A diet high in _____, but not one high in _____, causes a rise in tryptophan in the brain.

13. Some of this research may be exploited by the popular
     _____ and by suppliers to health-food
     _____.

14. Probably people can achieve a beneficial effect safely by
     drinking a cup of _____ _____ at bedtime and
     having a diet adequate in both protein and
     _____.

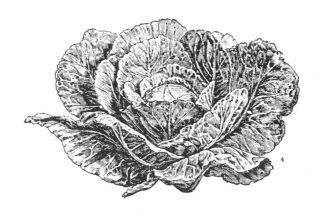

ANSWERS

1.   does
2.   liver
3.   twice
4.   blood
5.   deficiency, short
6.   neurotransmitters
7.   intriguing
8.   synapse
9.   inhibit
10.   norepinephrine
11.   tryptophan, depression
12.   carbohydrate, protein
13.   press, stores
14.   warm milk, carbohydrate

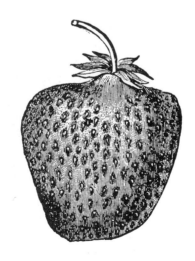

SELF TEST

1. Protein is composed of:
    a. carbon, hydrogen.
    b. carbon, hydrogen, oxygen.
    c. carbon, hydrogen, oxygen, nitrogen.
    d. sulfur, hydrogen, oxygen.
    e. sulfur, hydrogen, oxygen, carbon.

2. In a protein, _____ different amino acids may appear:
    a. 10
    b. 20
    c. 22
    d. 25
    e. 30

3. There are _____ amino acids essential for adults.
    a. 8
    b. 10
    c. 12
    d. 14
    e. 16

4. When two amino acids condense, the resulting structure is
    called a:
    a. polypeptide.
    b. dipeptide.
    c. tripeptide.
    d. condensation product.
    e. oligopeptide.

5. The bond between amino acids is a:
    a.   spearmint bond.
    b.   peptide bond.
    c.   hydropeptide bond.
    d.   hydrophobic bond.
    e.   tripeptide bond.

6. What is it called when three amino acids are bonded
    together by peptide bonds?
    a.   spearmint bond.
    b.   peptide bond.
    c.   hydropeptide bond.
    d.   hydrophobic bond.
    e.   tripeptide bond.

7. When many amino acids are bonded together, the resulting
    structure is called a/an:
    a.   oligopeptide.
    b.   tripetpide.
    c.   peptide.
    d.   polypeptide.

8. A complete protein is:
    a.   a protein containing all the amino acids in
         human nutrition.
    b.   one or more complex tangled chains of amino acids.
    c.   a simple structure comprised of 22 amino acids
         arranged in a geometric pattern.
    d.   an aggregate of carbon, hydrogen, and oxygen atoms.

9. The change in a protein's shape brought about by heat,
    acid, or other conditions is known as:
    a.   denaturation.
    b.   renaturation.
    c.   regeneration.
    d.   degeneration.

10. Enzymes are made of:
     a.   carbohydrate.
     b.   fat.
     c.   protein.
     d.   glucose.

11. A protein catalyst is:
     a.   a vitamin.
     b.   an enzyme.
     c.   a molecule.
     d.   a synthetic hormone.

12. The amino acid essential for infants, but not for adults, is:
    a. glycine.
    b. serine.
    c. histidine.
    d. tryptophan.
    e. valine.

13. (If your instructor wishes you to memorize the eight essential amino acids, you can practice here:
    T _____   T _____   P_____
    V_____   I_____   M_____
                          L _____
                          L_____

14. A measure of the unused amino acids from protein is:
    a. the amount of urea excreted.
    b. lack of growth.
    c. excretion of nitrogen.
    d. sulfur breath.

15. The reference protein is:
    a. egg protein.
    b. milk protein.
    c. meat.
    d. muscle meat without fat.

16. All but one of the following is a means of measuring protein quality:
    a. comparison with a reference protein.
    b. chemical scoring.
    c. biological value.
    d. growth coefficient.
    e. net protein utilization.

17. PER is:
    a. a ratio of protein efficiency.
    b. an abbreviation for percent to determine how much protein is in a diet.
    c. the Latin abbreviation for protein.

18. Animal proteins are generally of higher quality than plant proteins.
    a. true
    b. false

19. The space between the cells is called the:
     a. intravascular space.
     b. intercellular space.
     c. interstitial space.
     d. intracellular space.
     e. b or c

20. Proteins include all but one of the following:
     a. antibodies.
     b. the substance that clots blood (fibrin).
     c. connective tissue (collagen).
     d. pigments in the retina of the eye (opsin).
     e. the sex hormones.

21. Roles of protein include all but one of the following:
     a. maintaining water balance.
     b. transporting nutrients and molecules.
     c. emulsifying fats to prepare them for digestion.
     d. helping to replace GI tract cells.
     e. carrying iron.

22. Malnutrition caused by outright starvation is called:
     a. kwashiorkor.
     b. marasmus.
     c. synergism.

23. Malnutrition caused by protein deficiency in the presence
     of adequate kcalories is called:
     a. kwashiorkor.
     b. marasmus.
     c. synergism.

24. Adult PCM is often associated with:
     a. alcoholism.
     b. diabetes.
     c. pancreatic disease.

25. Adult kwashiorkor can occur in:
     a. alcoholics.
     b. hospital patients.
     c. anorexia nervosa.
     d. a and b
     e. a, b, and c

26. - 30 Indicate the nitrogen balance to be expected in the following individuals:
a. negative.   b. positive.   c. equilibrium.

_____ 26. A growing child.
_____ 27. A pregnant woman.
_____ 28. A lactating mother.
_____ 29. A sick person confined to bed.
_____ 30. A college student who gets an A in nutrition.

31. The Dietary Goals suggest _____ that the percent of your total kcalories from protein be:
a. 10-15%.
b. 15-25%.
c. 50%.
d. 5-10%.

32. If a person consumes too much protein, any of the following except one might be a possibility:
a. hypertrophy of the liver.
b. kidney growing too large.
c. dehydration.
d. crowding out of other nutritious foods.
e. weight loss.

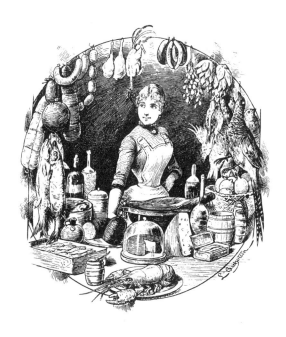

ANSWERS

1.   c
2.   c
3.   a
4.   b
5.   b
6.   e
7.   d
8.   a
9.   a
10.   c
11.   b
12.   c
13.   see below
14.   a
15.   a
16.   d
17.   a
18.   a
19.   b
20.   e
21.   c
22.   b
23.   a
24.   a
25.   d
26.   b
27.   b
28.   c
29.   a
30.   c
31.   a
32.   e

13.   T hreonine
      V aline
                    T ryptophan
                    I soleucine
                    L eucine
                    L ysine
                              P henylalanine
                              M ethionine

RECIPES YOU CAN TRY...

"PROTEIN" FOR BREAKFAST

Studies show that breakfast is the most neglected meal of the day. Few people realize how much they are depriving themselves by not eating breakfast, **or** by eating the wrong foods (such as sugars or simple starches).

<u>Why is breakfast important?</u>

You have been fasting usually for about ten hours. Your blood sugar level is low or on the verge of dropping and this slows your reactions and thinking. Energy levels are low. School achievement is poor for students, tempers are short, and much of the zest for life is missing because <u>your blood sugar determines how you think and act and feel</u> during the day.

Also, if the morning meal is neglected, it is very hard to obtain enough nutrients from lunch and dinner to provide the recommended daily allowances of nutrients.

<u>Breakfast Alternatives</u>: (Also include juice or fruit).

1. Place a fried or poached egg on a flour tortilla, melt cheese over the top.
2. Hamburger patty or fish sticks with or without cheese.
3. Sandwiches:
    a. One with meat will provide protein, iron, thiamin, riboflavin, and niacin.
    b. Cheese with bacon, ham or lunchmeat.
    c. Fried eggs and luncheon meat or frankfurters served on a bun.
    d. Scrambled eggs on bread, sprinkled with cheddar cheese, chives, Parmesan.
    e. Cottage cheese on whole wheat toast.
4. Deviled eggs.
5. Cheese souffle.
6. Rice pudding or custard.
7. Yogurt, fruit, and toast.
8. Bean soup or bean burrito.

9. Cottage cheese and applesauce or other fruit.
10. Leftover macaroni and cheese, leftover sliced meat, chicken, etc.
11. Breakfast yogurt "sundaes" with favorite fresh or dried fruit or nut toppings. (Important: Use plain yogurt, fruit-flavored yogurts are too sugary).

Breakfast Beverages: (Use blender or beater).

1. Combine and blend orange juice, milk, and a banana with egg.
2. Combine milk, lo-cal preserves, and egg.
3. Combine pineapple juice, banana, and egg.

Yogurt, dry milk powder, fruits, juices, and flavorings can be used.
EXAMPLE: 3/4 cup orange juice, 1 small carrot (sliced), 1/2 banana, 1 egg, 1/3 cup dry milk, 1 tsp honey.

HOMEMADE GRANOLA

Small box rolled oats
1 cup shredded coconut (unsweetened)
1 cup favorite nuts and seeds (almonds, sliced cashews, whole sunflower seeds--hulled).
1 cup raw wheat germ (be sure it is fresh)
    Mix together all dry ingredients

In another bowl: Mix 3/4 cup safflower oil, 1/3 cup water, 1½ tsp vanilla extract, 1½ tsp salt, 3/4 cup honey, 2 tsp of cinnamon. Mix this mixture thoroughly with a whip or hand beater, or use blender. The honey helps mix the oil and water together.

Pour the oil mixture into the oats mixture and mix with hands until evenly damp. Spread mix about ½ inch thick on oiled cookie or baking sheets, or broiler pan. Place these in slow oven (250°) from 1 to 1½ hours. Turn mixture with spatula after the first half hour and again every 15 minutes until oats are light golden brown. Remove from oven and turn mixture again. Let cool and add 1 cup raisins or other dried fruits. Store in a tightly-closed container in a cool place.

CHAPTER 5
Digestion, Absorption, and Transport

YOU WILL LEARN...

1. The problems of digestion, and how they are solved by the body.

2. The anatomy of the digestive tract.

3. The process of digestion and how the body deals with carbohydrate, fat, and protein.

4. Where the six nutrients are digested and absorbed and what happens to fiber.

5. How absorption of the digested nutrients takes place.

6. Why predigested protein is of no benefit.

7. The facts about food combinations.

8. How absorbed nutrients are released into the blood or lymph.

9. The special arrangement the body makes for fats.

10. What chylomicrons are.

11. The anatomy of the circulatory, vascular, and lymphatic systems.

12. The important differences between VLDL, LDL, and HDL.

13. How cholesterol is excreted with fiber, and the important difference between bran, pectin, and other fibers.

14. How to make your digestive system work well for you.

DIGESTION, ABSORPTION, AND TRANSPORT

THE PROBLEMS OF DIGESTION

1. Some of the same passages used for air are used for food, and we don't want food or liquid in the _____.

2. Food has to go through the _____ to get to the stomach.

3. The food must be ground up and mixed with _____.

4. Food must be finely divided and suspended in a water solution so that every particle is available to the digestive _____.

5. The material in the digestive tract must keep moving slowly but steadily, with ways of eliminating _____ or infection.

6. The enzymes must digest food without digesting the _____ itself.

7. Waste matter needs to be _____ periodically.

ANATOMY OF THE DIGESTIVE TRACT

8. The gastrointestinal tract, called _____ for short, is also referred to as the _____ canal.

CHAPTER 5: DIGESTION, ABSORPTION, AND TRANSPORT

REVIEW THE MINIGLOSSARY OF GI TERMS SO THAT YOU WILL BE FAMILIAR WITH THE VOCABULARY USED IN THE REMAINING PART OF THIS CHAPTER.

REVIEW THE ROUTE FOLLOWED BY NUTRIENTS FROM MOUTH TO ANUS, THE INVOLUNTARY MUSCLES, AND THE GLANDS.

9. Glands that secrete materials "out" into the digestive tract, or on to the skin (like sweat) are called _____ glands.

10. Glands that secrete "in" (into the blood) are called _____ glands.

11. After a mouthful of food has been swallowed, it is called a _____.

12. The successive waves of involuntary contraction passing along the walls of the intestine are called _____.

13. Special muscles that contract tightly, called _____ muscles, divide the tract into its principal divisions.

14. Liquefying food by physical action takes place in the _____ and _____.

15. When the mixture is churned and has gastric juices added, it is called _____, and is expelled into the duodenum.

THE PROCESS OF DIGESTION

16. No matter what your diet, all foods are basically composed of building blocks of _____, _____, and _____.

17. Five different body organs secrete digestive juices: the salivary glands, the stomach, the small intestine, the liver, and the _____.

18. The digestion of starch begins in your mouth with salivary _____. (An older name for this substance is ptyalin.)

19. No other nutrient is acted upon in the mouth but _____ is added.

20. The gastric juice is kept from digesting the stomach itself because of the thick lining of _____.

21. Strong acidity of the stomach is _____ (desirable/not desirable) and taking antacids does not solve the problems of overeating or of not chewing food properly.

22. The digestion of starch gradually ceases as the stomach _____ penetrates the bolus.

23. The major digestive event in the stomach is the _____ of proteins. The enzyme _____ works as a catalyst along with the gastric juice.

24. There is minor action in the stomach on carbohydrates, fat, and _____, but none on _____.

25. Most of the digestion takes place in the small intestine where three more _____ _____ are contributed.

26. Glands in the intestinal wall secrete a watery juice containing all three kinds of digestive enzymes--carbohydrases, lipases, and _____, and others as well.

27. The secretion of the intestinal glands, _____ _____, contains enzymes for the digestion of carbohydrate and protein and a minor enzyme for fat digestion.

28. The exocrine secretion of the pancreas, _____ juice, containing enzymes for the digestion of carbohydrate, fat and protein, flows through the _____ duct.

29. An endocrine function of the pancreas is the secretion of _____ and other hormones.

30. The pancreatic and bile ducts conduct pancreatic and liver secretions into the _____ _____.

31. There are _____ sets of enzymes to digest each of the energy nutrients.

32. When the pancreas fails, however, _____ digestion is seriously impaired.

33. Pancreatic juice also contains _____ _____ to neutralize the acidic chyme as it enters the small intestine.

34. The contents of the digestive tract, after entering the small intestine, are kept neutral or slightly _____.

35. The liver secretes _____ continuously, but it is stored in the _____ and not released into the intestine until fat is present for emulsification.

36. All the energy nutrients are digested in the _____ _____.

37. Most proteins are broken down to dipeptides, tripeptides and _____ _____ before they are absorbed.

38. The small intestine, being neutral, permits the growth of _____.

39. Vitamin _____, biotin and other B vitamins are produced by intestinal bacteria. These bacteria are known as the _____ _____.

40. Vitamins, minerals, and water are mostly _____ as is.

41. Still remaining in the digestive tract is _____.

42. Functions of fiber include retaining water, keeping the stools soft, and carrying out of the body excess fat, sterols, and _____ _____. Actually, some of the fiber is broken down to simpler compounds by the intestinal _____.

43. The conservative body recycles much material, especially water and dissolved _____.

THE PROBLEMS OF ABSORPTION

44. The twenty feet of small intestine actually provide a surface area whose extent is greater than a _____ of a football field for nutrient molecules to be absorbed.

45. Fluids continually _____ the undersides of these surfaces to wash away absorbed nutrients to their destinations.

CHAPTER 5: DIGESTION, ABSORPTION, AND TRANSPORT

ANATOMY OF THE ABSORPTIVE SYSTEM

46. The small intestine is a tube about _____ feet long and an _____ or so across. Its inner surface is wrinkled into hundreds of _____.

47. Each of these folds is covered with thousands of projections called _____. A single _____ is composed of hundreds of cells and is covered with its own microscopic hairs, the _____.

48. The hairlike _____ trap nutrient molecules, and can digest them further, if necessary.

49. There are two transport systems ready for nutrients absorbed into the cells, the _____ and the _____ system.

50. Lymph is the body's _____ fluid. It squishes around in a system of vessels and ducts known as the _____ system.

Closer Look at the Intestinal Cells

51. The enzymes and "pumps" lying within the microvilli recognize and act on different _____.

52. Digestion and absorption are very well _____ by the body.

53. Predigested protein is not as well absorbed by the body as whole protein because there is no coordination of digestion and _____.

54. Because of the lack of protein carriers, amino acids arriving in mass cannot be absorbed and can cause discomfort, cramping, nausea, and _____.

55. Because specific amino acids share these carriers, too many of one and not enough of the other can cause not only competition but a _____, thus reducing the total supply of usable protein.

56. Amino acid supplementation in combination with poor quality proteins, however, can provide a _____ closer to what the body needs.

57. An understanding of the digestive system enables one to evaluate ideas such as "food combining." Sugars and proteins eaten together, or within four hours of one another, may promote better retention of the _____.

NOTE TO STUDENT : The beauty of nature's plan can be appreciated and respected. We can't change the plan, and we can best cooperate with it by providing a variety of well-selected foods rather than trying to live on vitamin pills and various "supplements." Also, we should not make the body's task difficult by choosing too many empty-kcalorie and manufactured "foods."

58. Each part of the intestinal tract is specialized for different absorptive functions. The top portion of the duodenum absorbs calcium and several B vitamins such as thiamin and _____.

59. The jejunum absorbs _____. Vitamin _____ is absorbed at the end of the ileum.

Release of Absorbed Nutrients

60. Water-soluble nutrients are released directly into the _____.

61. Larger lipids and fat-soluble vitamins, triglycerides, cholesterol, and phospholipids are wrapped in protein coats as _____ and then released into the _____ system.

IF NECESSARY, REVIEW TRANSPORT OF NUTRIENTS INTO BLOOD, ANATOMY OF THE CIRCULATORY SYSTEM

62. A nutrient entering the bloodstream or lymphatic system may then be transported to any of the _____ _____.

The Vascular System

63. The vascular system is a closed system of vessels through which blood flows continuously in a figure eight, with the heart serving as a pump at the _____ _____.

See Figure 5

64. A vessel carrying blood away from the heart is an _____. A small vessel branching from an artery is a _____ and a vessel carrying blood back to the heart is a _____.

65. There is something different about the routing of the blood past the digestive system, however. Blood leaving the digestive system goes by way of a vein to the _____ instead of to the heart.

66. The blood arriving at the intestines flows through the _____, a strong, flexible membrane that supports the abdominal organs.

67. The vein collecting blood from the mesentery and conducting it to the liver is the _____ vein.

68. The vein collecting blood from the liver, returning it to the heart is the _____ vein.

69. The body's major metabolic organ is the _____.

70. Poison from barbiturates, alcohol, mercury, or hepatitis damages the _____ as it accumulates and attempts to metabolize these. Thus, the liver protects the heart and brain.

The Lymphatic System

71. The lymphatic system is similar to the water-filled spaces in a _____.

72. The lymph fluid is almost like blood except it has no _____ _____ cells.

73. Nutrients that are first absorbed into lymph soon get into the _____.

74. The duct that conveys lymph toward the heart is the _____-duct.

TRANSPORT OF LIPIDS: LIPOPROTEINS

75. In the circulatory systems, lipids always travel from place to place wrapped in _____ coats, that is, as _____.

CHAPTER 5: DIGESTION, ABSORPTION, AND TRANSPORT

76. Newly absorbed lipids leaving the intestinal cells are mostly packaged in the lipoproteins known as _____.

77. Lipids that have been processed or made in the liver are released in lipoproteins known as _____ and _____.

78. Lipids returning to the liver from other parts of the body are packaged in lipoproteins known as _____.

79. Lipoproteins are different in their _____ and density.

80. There are important health implications for HDL and _____.

81. Raised _____ concentrations are associated with an increased risk of heart attack.

82. Raised _____ concentrations are associated with a <u>low</u> risk of heart attack.

Chylomicrons: From the Intestinal Cells

83. Chylomicrons are large, fluffy _____ that float at the top of a sample of blood. They are dismantled by the liver within 14 hours or _____ and new lipids for use by other body cells are made.

VLDL and LDL: From the Liver

84. The liver cells rearrange most of the triglycerides from the _____. Other fatty acids, _____, and other compounds are made. More lipids may be made from _____.

85. Some of these excess lipids either need to be stored or used. To transport them, the liver once again wraps them in proteins--this time as VLDL and _____.

86. VLDL stands for very low _____ lipoprotein. It is also called "pre-beta" lipoprotein.

87. LDL, low density lipoprotein, is also called "_____ lipoprotein."

88. HDL and LDL contain more cholesterol than _____. They are smaller and denser.

89.   The body cells can select fat from these particles for many important uses, or _____ them for later use.

HDL: From the Body Cells

90.   HDL stands for _____ density lipoprotein.

91.   When the cells mobilize fat from storage, most of the triglycerides are used for _____, and the cells return the unused _____ and phospholipids to the blood.

92.   The packages in which unused fats are found are the _____.

93.   It is believed that the function of HDL is return to the liver for _____ or disposal. HDLs are also called "alpha" _____.

Atherosclerosis and the Lipoproteins

94.   Because lipoproteins contain clues to the risks of heart and artery disease, scientists now use the term _____ instead of "hyperlipidemia" in order to recognize the carrier in which the lipid appears.

95.   The cholesterol deposited in the artery wall plaques is carried mostly by the _____. High blood cholesterol reflects a high _____ concentration.

96.   It is not useful to only measure the amount of cholesterol in the blood; it is necessary to know whether it is contained in LDL or _____.

97.   Raised _____ concentrations represent lower total body cholesterol and a lower risk of developing atherosclerosis or a heart attack.

NOTE TO STUDENT;   IN STUDYING FOR AN EXAMINATION, THINK OF THE HDLS AS THE "GOOD GUYS", THE LDLS AS THE "BAD GUYS."

98.   Some people have lipid profiles high in chylomicrons, VLDL, or LDL for _____ reasons; others have similar profiles from poor _____ habits.

99.   Three ways of controlling blood cholesterol levels include:
       1.   Controlling weight,
       2.   Eating less saturated fat,
       3.   _____ intensely and frequently.

Excretion of Cholesterol with Fiber

100.   Cholesterol is used by the _____ to manufacture _____.

101.   When emulsified fat is absorbed, some of the _____ goes with it.

102.   The enterohepatic circulation of bile indicates the path of bile from liver, to gallbladder, to intestine and back to the _____.

103.   Bile that is left in the intestine travels down the GI tract and is excreted from the body with other _____ material.

104.   Fibers that lower blood cholesterol include _____ and hemicellulose, but not _____ bran.

105.   Foods, not _____ nutrients, offer the greatest benefits to health.

THE SYSTEM AT ITS BEST

106.   Good health of the G.I. tract is promoted by factors of lifestyle such as sleep, exercise, and _____ of mind. It helps to be relaxed and _____ at mealtimes.

107.   Another factor is your _____. Balance, variety, adequacy and _____ are helpful.

108.   Almost every nutrient depends on every _____ nutrient.

SUMMING UP

Review Text if Necessary

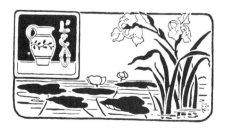

ANSWERS

1. lungs
2. diaphragm
3. water
4. enzymes
5. poison
6. stomach
7. excreted
8. G. I., alimentary
9. exocrine
10. endocrine
11. bolus
12. peristalsis
13. sphincter
14. mouth, stomach
15. chyme
16. carbohydrate, fat, protein
17. pancreas
18. amylase
19. water
20. mucus
21. desirable
22. acid
23. hydrolysis, pepsin
24. protein, minerals
25. digestive juices
26. proteases
27. intestinal juice
28. pancreatic, pancreatic
29. insulin
30. small intestine
31. two
32. fat
33. sodium bicarbonate
34. alkaline
35. bile, gallbladder
36. small intestine
37. amino acids
38. bacteria
39. k, intestinal flora
40. absorbable
41. fiber
42. bile acids, bacteria
43. salts
44. quarter
45. bathe
46. 20, inch, folds
47. villi, villus, microvilli
48. microvilli

49. bloodstream, lymphatic
50. interstitial, lymphatic
51. nutrients
52. coordinated
53. absorption
54. diarrhea
55. deficiency
56. balance
57. protein
58. riboflavin
59. triglycerides, B12
60. blood
61. lipoproteins, lymphatic
62. body cells
63. crossover point
64. artery, capillary, vein
65. liver
66. mesentery
67. portal
68. hepatic
69. liver
70. liver
71. sponge
72. red blood
73. blood
74. thoracic
75. protein, lipoproteins
76. chylomicrons
77. VLDL, LDL
78. HDL
79. size
80. LDL
81. LDL
82. HDL
83. particles, less
84. chylomicrons, cholesterol, carbohydrates
85. LDL
86. density
87. beta
88. chylomicrons
89. store
90. high
91. energy, cholesterol
92. HDL
93. recycling, lipoproteins
94. hyperlipoproteinemia
95. LDL,LDL
96. HDL
97. HDL

98. genetic, health
99. Exercising
100. liver, bile
101. bile
102. liver
103. waste
104. pectin, wheat
105. purified
106. state, tranquil
107. diet, moderation
108. other

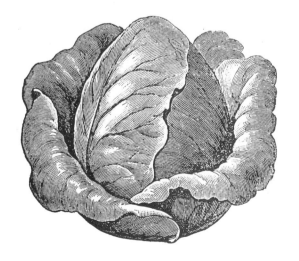

HIGHLIGHT 5:   STRESS AND NUTRITION

1. Stress can be anything that you experience as a threat to your stability or _____.

2. The stress response is the body's way of responding to such a perceived _____.

3. The body's response to stress begins with an _____ -reaction, proceeds through resistance, and then either recovery or _____.

The Stress Response

4. The body responds to the stress of an alarm signal:
    a. eyes widen.
    b. muscles tense.
    c. breathing quickens.
    d. heart races.
    e. liver releases glucose.
    f. fat cells release fatty acids and ketones.
    g. body protein breaks down.
    h. blood vessels in muscles expand.
    i. the GI tract blood vessels constrict.
    j. GI tract glands shut down.
    k. less blood flows to the kidney.
    l. less blood flows to the skin.
    m. blood clots faster.
    n. hearing gets sharper.
    o. hair may stand on end.
    p. the brain produces a substance to dull _____.

Body Reserves Drawn on During Stress

5. One mineral that is lost rather quickly is _____.

6. After a day of fasting, the only significant continuing glucose supply comes from body _____.

7. Another important nutrient lost from the body during stress is _____ from the bones.

Nutrition Prior to Periods of Stress

8. Protein and calcium are important to eat, but it is equally important to _____.

9. It is poor advice to someone under severe stress to tell them to eat. They _____ or if they can, they can't _____ what they've eaten.

10. Fasting is itself a _____ on the body.

11. The depletion of nutrients during stress includes all the vitamins and _____ that are not stored in the body.

12. Multivitamin- _____ preparations might be needed in amounts comparable to the _____ for people under stress who are not eating much.

Stress Eating

13. The _____ of eating helps to relieve _____.

14. Eating or the food eaten may lead to the release of internal _____. One needs to substitute _____, listening to music, or other restful activities.

Nutrition in the Recovery Period

15. Replenish depleted nutrient _____.

16. If you have lost weight, _____ it back.

17. If you have gained weight, diet and _____.

18. Build up mental fitness so the next stressful event will not be _____.

Stress Management

19. Change how you _____ the stressful event so you will not react violently.

20. Learn to express yourself, or to _____ your feelings.

21. Take time _____ for relaxation and exercise.

22. Expand your _____ support system.

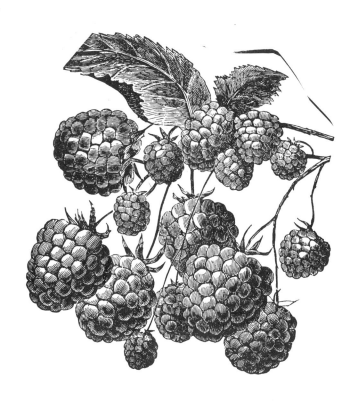

ANSWERS

1. equilibrium
2. threat
3. alarm, exhaustion
4. pain
5. potassium
6. protein
7. calcium
8. exercise
9. can't, assimilate
10. stress
11. minerals
12. mineral, RDA
13. behavior, stress
14. tranquilizers, meditation
15. stores
16. gain
17. exercise
18. overwhelming
19. perceive
20. ventilate
21. out
22. social

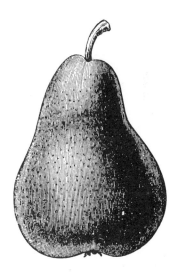

SELF TEST

1. The three segments of the small intestine are:
    a. the trachea, the esophagus, and the cardiac sphincter.
    b. the duodenum, the jejunum, and the ileum.
    c. the pylorus, the esophagus, and the jejunum.
    d. the jejunum, the appendix, and the ileum.

2. A gland that secretes its materials <u>into</u> the blood is
    called an _____ gland.
    a. exocrine.
    b. endocrine.
    c. esophagus.
    d. exitcrine.

3. A gland that secretes its materials "out" is called an
    _____ gland.
    a. exocrine.
    b. endocrine.
    c. exitcrine.
    d. esoteric.

4. The muscular action that pushes food along the entire GI
    tract is called:
    a. homeostasis.
    b. segmentation.
    c. peristalsis.

5. After a mouthful of food is swallowed, it is called:
    a. a cud.
    b. a chew.
    c. a bolus.
    d. chyme.

6. When liquefied food leaves the stomach through the pylorus, it is called:
    a. kime.
    b. chyme.
    c. amylase.
    d. chyle.

7. Gastric juice contains water, enzymes, and:
    a. mucus.
    b. hydrochloric acid.
    c. lipase.

8. The major digestive event in the stomach is the:
    a. digestion of proteins.
    b. hydrolysis of proteins.
    c. digestion of starch.
    d. hydrolysis of starch and protein.
    c. digestion of fat.

9. Bile is:
    a. an enzyme.
    b. an emulsifier.
    c. a secretion of the liver.
    d. a and b
    e. b and c

10. Some proteins you eat will act as enzymes in the body.
    a. true
    b. false

11. Which of the following are <u>not</u> absorbed in the small intestine:
    a. fat and carbohydrate.
    b. protein and vitamins.
    c. water and fiber.
    d. minerals and vitamins.

12. The absorptive system of the human body provides a large surface where the nutrient molecules can make contact and be absorbed. This total area is approximately:
    a. 1/4 acre.
    b. 20 feet.
    c. 1/2 acre.
    d. 40 square feet.

13. The finger-like projections from the folds of the small
     intestine are called:
     a. microvilli.
     b. villi.
     c. lymphatic nodes.
     d. digestive nodules.

14. The body's interstitial fluid is called:
     a. blood.
     b. water.
     c. cellular fluid.
     d. lymph.
     e. saline solution.

15. Which would be best absorbed and utilized by the body,
     especially by a weakened individual:
     a. a hydrolyzed amino acid preparation.
     b. liquid protein.
     c. whole protein.

16. Which statement is most nearly correct about food
     combining?
     a. It represents a gross underestimation of the
         body's capabilities.
     b. It ensures that each nutrient will be digested
         completely without competition from another.
     c. It keeps the stomach from being overloaded.
     d. It is a wise course to follow for improved health.

17. Water-soluble nutrients are released from the small
     intestine directly into the:
     a. lymph.
     b. bloodstream.
     c. large intestine.
     d. heart.

18. Chylomicrons are released into the:
     a. blood.
     b. lymph.
     c. liver.
     d. intestine.

19. A vessel carrying blood away from the heart is called:
     a. an artery.
     b. a capillary.
     c. a vein.

20. A vessel carrying blood back to the heart is called:
     a. an artery.
     b. a capillary.
     c. a vein.

21. The strong, flexible membrane that surrounds and supports
     the abdominal organs is called:
     a. the liver.
     b. the mesentery.
     c. the placenta.
     d. the portal membrane.

22. Drugs, alcohol, poison, and some viruses are screened from
     the body by:
     a. the intestinal cells.
     b. the brain.
     c. the liver.

23. Lymph contains everything that blood contains except :
     a. protoplasm.
     b. white blood cells.
     c. red blood cells.
     d. nutrient-transporting molecules.

24. When lipids are wrapped by the liver for transport in the
     blood, they are called:
     a. protein carriers.
     b. chylomicrons.
     c. lipoproteins.
     d. triglycerides.

25. All but one of the following are names of lipoproteins:
     a. VLDL.
     b. LDL.
     c. chylomicrons.
     d. HDL.
     e. FLDL.

26. Raised LDL levels indicate a _____ of heart
     attack.
     a. high risk
     b. low risk

27. Raised HDL levels indicate a _____ of heart
     attack.
     a. high risk
     b. low risk

28. Triglycerides comprise about _____ percent of dietary fat.
    a. five
    b. ninety-five
    c. fifty
    d. twenty-five

29. Lipids sent out from the liver are called:
    a. VLDL and LDL.
    b. LDL.
    c. HDL.
    d. chylomicrons.

30. Lipids sent out from the intestinal cells are called:
    a. VLDL and LDL.
    b. LDL.
    c. HDL.
    d. chylomicrons.

31. Lipids coming from the body cells (stored fat) are called:
    a. VLDL and LDL.
    b. LDL.
    c. HDL.
    d. chylomicrons.

32. The lipoproteins that carry the most cholesterol are the:
    a. HDL.
    b. LDL.
    c. RDA.
    d. HLD.

33. Abnormal lipid profiles can be caused by:
    a. genetic abnormalities.
    b. poor health habits.
    c. eating too much fiber.
    d. a and b
    e. b and c

34. Cholesterol is used by the liver to:
    a. screen out poisons.
    b. transport lipids.
    c. transport nutrients.
    d. manufacture bile.

35. Bile left in the intestine after emulsifying fat may be:
    a. recycled.
    b. excreted from the body.
    c. changed to LDL.
    d. a and b

36. The fiber that lowers blood cholesterol is:
     a. wheat fiber.
     b. pectin.
     c. hemicellulose.
     d. b and c

HIGHLIGHT 5

37. Examples of stress are:
     a. eating sugar.
     b. walking in the cold.
     c. getting a promotion.
     d. being frightened.
     e. all of the above

38. Which of the following is <u>not</u> a response to stress?
     a. eyes narrow
     b. muscles tense
     c. fat cells release fatty acids and ketones
     d. protein tissue breaks down
     e. brain produces opium-like substance

39. One of the minerals most needed during stress is:
     a. vitamin C.
     b. iodine.
     c. potassium.
     d. chlorine.
     e. magnesium.

40. The energy nutrient most needed to prepare for stress is:
     a. fat.
     b. protein.
     c. carbohydrate.

41. All people lose weight in response to stress.
     a. True
     b. False

42. Internal tranquilizers are:
  a. subordinate antistressors.
  b. subliminal easers.
  c. endogenous opiates.
  d. narcotics.
  e. soporifics.

43. To have strong bones and healthy muscles one needs to:
  a. eat a surplus of needed nutrients.
  b. exercise regularly.
  c. think positively.
  d. b and c.
  e. a, b, and c.

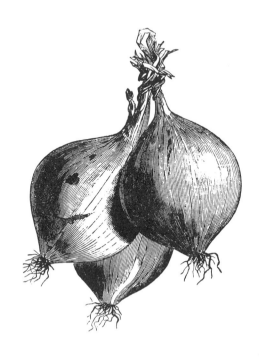

ANSWERS

```
 1.    b
 2.    b
 3.    a
 4.    c
 5.    c
 6.    b
 7.    b
 8.    b
 9.    e
10.    b
11.    c
12.    a
13.    b
14.    d
15.    c
16.    a
17.    b
18.    b
19.    a
20.    c
21.    b
22.    c
23.    c
24.    c
25.    e
26.    a
27.    b
28.    b
29.    a
30.    d
31.    c
32.    b
33.    d
34.    d
35.    d
36.    d
37.    e
38.    c
39.    c
40.    b
41.    b
42.    c
43.    b
```

COTTAGE CHEESE SCALLOPED POTATOES

This recipe is recommended for its ease of digestion, flavor, fine protein, and economy.

    1 cup thinly sliced raw potatoes
    1 cup creamed cottage cheese
    1/2 tbsp butter
    1/2 cup milk (about)
    salt and pepper to taste

Butter a small baking dish. Arrange alternate layers of seasoned potatoes and cottage cheese. Pour on milk to cover potatoes. Bake in moderate oven, 325-350°, about 45 minutes or until potatoes are tender. The baking time may be shortened by heating the milk before adding it to the potatoes. Makes 2 generous servings.

Serve with: Green cabbage or another green vegetable, ginger-bread or muffins, fruit, and milk.

BRAN MUFFINS

Here is a fine way to include more fiber in your diet.

1-1/2 cups bran or bran cereal	1/2 cup raisins, dates
1/2 cup boiling water	or prunes
1 egg, slightly beaten	1-1/4 tsp soda
1 cup buttermilk	1/4 tsp. salt
1/4 cup salad oil	1-1/4 cups flour

In a mixing bowl, mix bran cereal with boiling water, stirring to moisten evenly. Set aside until cool, then add egg, buttermilk, oil and fruit and blend well. Stir together the soda, salt, sugar, and flour, then stir into bran mixture. Spoon batter into buttered muffin cups, filling 2/3 to 3/4 full. Bake in a 425° oven for 20 minutes or until tops spring back when lightly touched. Serve hot or rewarm. Makes 12-14 muffins. Extras freeze well.

VERY EASY CHOWDER

1 small onion
2 tbsp butter
2 potatoes
1 can minced clams, and juice
1-1/2 cups milk
salt, pepper, paprika

Saute a chopped small onion in butter; add raw, peeled, diced potatoes and 1/2 cup water. Cover and cook until potato is tender. Add clams, juice, milk, and seasonings. Heat to boiling. Serve with oyster crackers if desired. Serves two or three.

This is a good recipe to have on hand for a cold day when you might have a guest and you may have the ingredients on hand without having to shop. It tastes so much better than the canned chowders! Add a crumbled slice of bacon for extra flavor.

POTATO SOUP

1 cup diced potatoes
1/2 cup diced celery
1/4 cup minced onion
3/4 cup water (about)

1 cup milk
1 tbsp butter
1 tsp salt
dash pepper

Cook potatoes, celery, and onion with salt in just enough water to barely cover. Cook 10-15 minutes over moderate heat until vegetables are tender. Mash vegetables slightly in liquid. Add milk and butter, heat. Add pepper and celery salt, if preferred. Makes 2 generous servings. Serve with whole wheat toast and a generous salad of fresh fruit and cottage cheese.

Make other delicious cream soups with leftover cooked vegetables such as spinach, peas, carrots, and corn. Use about 1/2 cup mashed vegetables to 1 cup milk; add seasoning and 1 tsp of butter.

CHAPTER 6

Metabolism: Feasting, Fasting, and Energy Balance

YOU WILL LEARN...

1. What metabolism is.

2. How different compounds are put together for use by the body.

3. How nutrients are broken down to use for energy or to reassemble into different compounds.

4. What happens to carbohydrate, protein and fat in the body.

5. How fasting affects the body.

6. Problems caused by popular low-carbohydrate diets.

7. What being in "ketosis" means.

8. How to estimate kcalories in food.

9. How to estimate kcalories burned in activities.

10. What the SDE for food is and how to calculate it.

11. What factors affect BMR.

12. How to recognize a realistic and effective diet plan.

HIGHLIGHT 6: NUTRITION FOR THE ATHLETE

13. How much protein an athlete really needs.

14. How to supply the kcalorie needs.

15. The truth about glycogen loading.

16. What the best pre-game meal consists of.

CHAPTER 6: METABOLISM

17. About athlete's liquid needs, and how to meet them.

18. The problems of athletes.

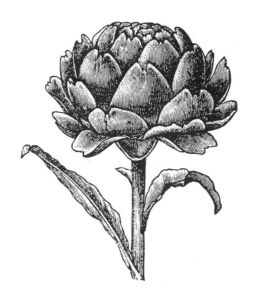

METABOLISM: FEASTING, FASTING, AND ENERGY BALANCE

1. Metabolism could be defined as the way the body handles the
   _____ _____.

2. The complete definition of metabolism is the sum total of
   all the _____ reactions that go on in living cells.

3. To follow carbohydrate through metabolism you can simply
   follow _____

4. To follow lipids through metabolism, you can follow
   _____ and _____ _____.

5. To follow protein through metabolism, you can follow
   _____.

BUILDING BODY COMPOUNDS

6. _____ is any reaction in which small molecules are
   put together to build large ones. Anabolic reactions
   involve reduction and <u>consume</u> energy.

7. _____ _____ may be strung together to make
   glycogen chains.

8. _____ _____ may be used to make proteins

9. _____ and fatty acids may be assembled into
   triglycerides.

BREAKING DOWN NUTRIENTS FOR ENERGY

10. _____ involves reactions in which large molecules
    are broken down to smaller ones. Catabolic reactions
    involve oxidation and <u>release</u> energy.

11. _____ in the liver cells do much of the body's
    catabolic work.

12. During metabolism the body actually separates the _____ of the digested energy nutrients from one another.

13. Learning how the atoms are separated, it is important to remember how many carbons are in the "_____" of their structures.

14. Glucose has ____ carbons, glycerol has ___. Fatty acids have multiples of _____ carbons, and amino acids have ____ or ____ or more with nitrogen attached. Three carbons can make glucose, two carbons cannot.

15. Pyruvate and pyruvic acid are the same because the ending "ate" is used interchangeably with the ending "_____."

16. The metabolic breakdown of glucose to pyruvate is called _____.

Glucose

17. In breaking down, glucose first splits in half, releasing _____.

18. The two identical halves resulting form this breakdown are both _____.

19. These halves could be put back together to form _____.

20. If the cell still needs energy, it could break the pyruvate molecules apart further by taking a carbon out of each one. The carbon combines with oxygen to make carbon _____ which soon is breathed out.

21. The 2-carbon compound remaining is acetate, called _____ CoA.

22. At this point the cell _____ (can/cannot) remake glucose.

23. One breathes harder during exercise because energy nutrients are being broken down to provide that energy, and _____ is ultimately involved in the oxidation process.

24. When acetyl CoA is split the released energy powers most of the cell's activities, and two more carbon _____ molecules are produced.

25. Review: the main steps in the metabolism of glucose are: glucose to _____ to _____ _____ to carbon _____. Only the first step is reversible.

26. The part of the process from acetyl COA to carbon dioxide is known as the _____ cycle.

27. Another name for TCA cycle is the _____ cycle.

28. Still another name associated with this for the same process is _____ phosphorylation.

29. Only the parts of protein and fat that can be converted to _____ can provied _____ for the body.

Glycerol and Fatty Acids

30. _____, under ordinary circumstances, cannot provide significant amounts of _____ for the brain and nervous systems.

31. Glycerol can yield glucose, but 3 out of 54 parts of the fat molecule represents only _____ % of its weight, so _____ % cannot be coverted to glucose at all.

Amino Acids

32. Ideally, amino acids will be used to replace needed _____ proteins.

33. If they are needed for energy, the _____ is removed and about _____ of the amino acids can be converted to pyruvate; the other half go either to acetyl _____ or directly into the _____ cycle.

34. The amino acids that can be used to make _____ can provide _____ for the body. About _____ percent of protein can be used for glucose when carbohydrate is not available.

35. The making of glucose from protein or from the glycerol protion of fat is called _____.

36. Protein can make you fat because it cannot be stored and has to be converted to other _____.

37. Excess protein is not a muscle-building food, it's a _____ -building food.

What Happens to the Nitrogen?

38. When you remove the nitrogen from protein, the process is called _____. The product is _____, chemically identical to the _____ in the bottled cleaning solutions.

39. Ammonia that is not used is quickly combined with a carbon-oxygen fragment to make _____.

40. Urea is the principal nitrogen-excretion product of _____.

41. One of the functions of the kidneys is to remove _____ from the blood for exretion in the _____.

42. The body's principal vehicle for excreting unused nitrogen is _____.

Putting it All Together

43. When all of the energy supplied from the last meal has been used up, and reserves of the various compounds are running low, its time to _____ again.

44. The average person consumes more than a _____ kcalories a year and expends more than _____ percent of them.

THE ECONOMY OF FEASTING

45. Metabolism favors _____ formation when you eat too much of any energy nutrient.

46. Surplus dietary fat will be routed to the assembly of _____ and stored in the fat cells.

47. Surplus protein will be converted to triglycerides and swell the _____ _____.

THE ECONOMY OF FASTING

48. Even when you are asleep, the cells of many organs are hard at work and spending _____.

49. What you do with your muscles during your waking hours represents about a _____ of the total energy you spend in one day.

50. If people choose not to eat, we say they are _____.

51. If they have no choice (as in a famine), we say they are _____.

52. There is no _____ difference between the two.

53. Normally the brain consumes about _____ of the total glucose used each day, about _____ to 600 calories' worth.

54. Body protein <u>always</u> breaks down to some extent during fasting in order to supply energy in the form of _____.

55. When the body extracts one molecule of glycerol from a triglyceride, the body disposes of 50-60 carbons' worth of fatty acids. If body protein would continue to break down as it does during the first few days of a fast, death would ensue within _____ weeks.

56. As the fast continues, the body adapts by producing an alternate energy source, _____.

57. Gradually ketone production rises until it meets about _____ of the brain's energy needs.

58. "Acetone breath" indicates that a person is in _____.

59. A ketone is a compound formed during the incomplete _____ of fatty _____. When their concentration rises, they spill into the _____.

60. The combination of high blood ketones and ketones in the urine is called _____.

61. A loss of appetite can be incurred by being in a state of ketosis <u>or</u> by following a low- _____ diet.

62. During fasting, _____ (more/less) fat is lost than on a low-kcalorie diet.

63. During fasting, weight loss may be dramatic, but _____ loss is less than when _____ food is supplied.

64. The physical symptoms of marasmus include wasting, slowed metabolism, lowered body temperature and _____ resistance to _____.

65. Some important body changes that take place in fasting are:
    a. sodium and _____ depletion
    b. an _____ in body uric acid
    c. a _____ in blood cholesterol
    d. a decrease in _____ hormone

The Low-Carbohydrate Diet

66. An economy similar to that of fasting prevails if a _____-carbohydrate diet is consumed.

67. The onset of _____ is always a signal that a _____ process has begun.

68. In a diet less than 900 kcalories it is pointless to provide _____ at all.

69. The person who wishes to lose body fat will select a balanced diet of _____ or more kcalories.

70. Most of the loss on a low-carbohydrate diet is from _____.

71. Learn to distinguish between loss of _____ and loss of weight.

The Protein-Sparing Fast

72. The ultimate criterion of success in any weight-loss program is maintenance of the new _____ weight.

73. The physicians originally experimenting with this diet used whole _____ _____ -rich foods.

74. When the diet was popularized, dieters drank "_____ _____" from low-quality sources.

75. Deaths were probably from _____ losses.

Moderate Weight Loss

76. The maximum rate that body fat breaks down is, for the average person, about _____ to _____ pounds per week.

77. A "low" kcalorie diet means living on food and
_____ _____.

78. One pound of body fat equals _____ kcal on oxidation.
However, a pound of pure fat would yield 4,086 kcal at
_____ kcal per gram.

ESTIMATION OF KCALOIRE INTAKE FROM FOOD

79. The bomb calorimeter measures kcalorie values by the
_____ given off or the amount of _____ consumed
in the burning.

80. The number of kcalories determined by direct calorimetry is
_____(higher/lower) than the number of
kcalories that same food could give to an animal.

81. The animal does not metabolize all the food all the way to
carbon _____ and water.

82. It you want to practice with food exchange calorie counts,
see if you can remember these seven values:

a cup skim milk _____ kcal
1/2 cup vegetable _____ kcal
1 portion fruit _____ kcal
1 portion bread or starchy vegetable _____ kcal
1 oz lean meat _____ kcal
1 tsp fat _____ kcal
1 tsp sugar _____ kcal

83. It may become more and more important to us to consider the
energy cost of food preparation and _____.

ESTIMATION OF KCALORIES OUTPUT BY THE BODY

84. One must also count energy _____.

Government Recommendations

85. Both the "reference" man and "reference" woman are
estimated to engage in _____ activity.

86. Older people need _____ kcalories, with the number
_____ about 10 percent per decade beyond age 30.

87. It is believed that for adults an _____ kcal range covers
most individuals.

CHAPTER 6: METABOLISM:

Diet Record Method

88. It is necessary to keep records for at least one _____ because intakes vary so much each day.

Laboratory Methods

89. _____ is always a by-product of energy expenditure.

90. Another indication for measuring energy expendure is the _____ consumed and carbon dioxide expelled, as this is in proportion to the heat released.

91. Human energy is spent in two major ways; on _____ and on voluntary _____.

92. Two-thirds of the energy spent in a day is for _____.

93. BMR is_____ (highest/lowest) in the young.

94. BMR is _____(higher-lower) in people with large surface areas.

95. BMR is _____(higher/lower) in females.

96. BMR _____ (increases/decreases) with age.

97. The real key to figuring BMR depends on _____ tissue or fat-free mass.

98. BMR _____ (increases/decreases) during a fever

99. Fasting and constant malnutrition _____ (lower/raise) the BMR.

100. The hormone secreted by the thryroid gland, regulating the basal metaboic rate is _____.

101. Mental activity requires _____ _____ energy.

102. The amount of energy used for an activity depends on body weight and _____.

103. The third component of energy expenditure has to do with processing _____. It is called SDE, or SDA.

Note to student: If you remember how many organs and cells are involved in digesting and absorbing food, it is easy to visualize the "cost" of this processing as approximately 10% of what is eaten.

104.   The specific _____effect, or specific _____activity of food needs to be added to the basic BMR figure in addition to energy expenditure for activity.

WEIGHT LOSS AND GAIN RATES

105.   A deficit of 500 kcal a day brings about loss of body fat at the rate of about _____ pound/s per week.

106.   Loss of body fat in excess of _____ pounds a week can rarely be sustained.

107.   A diet supplying fewer than _____ kcal per day is inadequate in vitamins and minerals.

108.   _____ and underweight are complex problems.

ANSWERS

1. energy nutrients
2. chemical
3. glucose
4. glycerol, fatty acids
5. amino acids
6. Anabolism
7. Glucose units
8. Amino acids
9. Glycerol
10. Catabolism
11. Enzymes
12. atoms
13. backbones
14. 6, 3, 2, 2, 3
15. 1c, acid
16. glycolysis
17. energy
18. pyruvate
19. glucose
20. dioxide
21. acetyl
22. cannot
23. oxygen
24. dioxide
25. pyruvate, acetyl CoA, dioxide
26. TCA
27. Krebs
28. oxidative
29. pyruvate, glucose
30. Fat, energy
31. 5, 95
32. body
33. nitrogen, half, CoA, TCA (or Krebs)
34. pyruvate, energy, 50
35. gluconeogenesis
36. compounds

37. fat
38 deamination, ammonia, ammonia
39. urea
40. metabolism
41. urea, urine
42. water
43. eat
44. million, 99
45. fat
46. triglycerides
47. fat cells
48. energy
49. third
50. fasting
51. starving
52. metabolic
53. two-thirds, 400
54. glucose
55. three
56. ketones
57. half
58. ketosis
59. oxidation, acids, urine
60. ketosis
61. kcalorie
62. less
63. fat, some
64. reduced, disease
65. a. potassium
     b. increase
     c. rise
     d. thyroid
66. low
67. ketosis, wasting
68. protein
69. 1200
70. water
71. fat
72. low
73. natural, protein
74. liquid protein
75. mineral
76. 1, 2
77. stored fat
78. 3,500, 9
79. heat, oxygen
80. higher
81. dioxide
82. 80, 25, 40, 70, 55, 45, 20

83. production
84. expenditure
85. light
86. fewer, decreasing
87. 800
88. week
89. Heat
90. oxygen
91. basal metabolism, activity
92. BMR
93. highest
94. higher
95. higher
96. decreases
97. lean
98. increases
99. lower
100. thyroxin
101. very little
102. time
103. food
104. dynamic, dynamic
105. one
106. two
107. 1,200
108. Obesity

HIGHLIGHT 6: NUTRITION FOR THE ATHLETE

NUTRITION FOR THE ATHLETE

1. Trainers often pass on much nutrition _____.

2. Despite nutrition information, tradition and superstition, the athlete often makes _____ food choices.

Protein Needs of Athletes

3. Athletes often believe that their diets should be extremely high in _____.

4. Actually, they probably use only _____ percent more protein that non-athletes.

5. The main concern is to eat enough protein-sparing kcalories to meet _____ needs. Athletes, then, need extra _____ not extra _____.

6. Building muscle requires _____ nitrogen balance.

7. Muscles only respond to the _____ placed upon them.

kCalorie Needs of Athletes

8. Athletes in active training average approximately _____ kcalories a day, sometimes even higher. It is almost impossible to eat this much nutrient-dense food in three meals; _____ to _____ meals make the task easier.

Gaining and Losing Weight

9. The most widespread nutrition-related abuse in sports is a high-_____ diet.

10. Further, the athlete must remember to cut _____ on calories between and after training periods.

11. Muscle turning to fat really means that _____ has been lost and _____ has been gained.

12. Abnormal heart rhythms have been seen in healthy adults after only _____ days of fasting.

13. Women athletes experience athletes' _____.

Energy for Muscle Work

14. Two-thirds of the body's glycogen is in the _____,and only _____ is in the liver to serve the rest of the body's needs.

15. After glucose has released its energy, only _____ and carbon-dioxide gas are left.

16. Athletes must condition their _____ and _____ systems with aerobic exercises rather than increasing muscle strength only.

17. Fat deposits supply energy for _____ but not for strenuous muscular work.

18. If muscles are in good shape, it is easier to keep off _____.

19. It takes _____ hours or more to restore muscle carbohydrate to its pre-exercise level after it has been completely exhausted.

20. Two pointers for the athlete in training are to:

    a. Take a periodic day's _____.
    b. Eat a _____ -rich diet.

21. Glycogen loading is not recommended more than about _____ times per year due to the effects on heart function.

22. Sometimes muscle and cardiac pain and _____ gain cancel the benefits of glycogen loading.

23. Specialists say it may be best to just eat a diet generally high in _____, and especially _____ before competition.

24. The winners watch all of the following to maximize performance:

    a. muscular conditioning
    b. aerobic (heart & lung) conditioning
    c. optimal iron and protein nutrition
    d. optimal _____ and _____ nutrition

The Pre-Game Meal

25. Olympic training tables are laden with _____.

26. Many athletes tolerate _____ meals best.

27. Any meal should be finished two to _____ hours before an event.

28. There is no ergogenic food or supplement. Ergogenic means _____ -producing.

The Athlete's Liquid Needs

29. Maintaining _____ balance is crucial to successful performance.

30. The first symptom of dehydration is _____.

31. A rapid water loss equal to 5 percent of body weight can reduce muscular work by _____ to _____ percent.

32. Salt tablets are/are not recommended.

33. Replacement of _____ and _____ may be more important than replacement of sodium.

34. Sweat replacers such as Gatorade are absorbed less/more rapidly than water.

35. Alcohol (as in beer) and caffeine (as in coffee) actually inhibit/promote water loss from the body.

Athletes' Anemia

36. Women athletes who are menstruating regularly may need an _____ supplement.

37. Some anemia may be an adaptation by the body to an _____ way of life.

ANSWERS

1. misinformation
2. poor
3. protein
4. ten
5. energy, carbohydrate, protein
6. positive
7. demands
8. 6,000, five, six
9. fat
10. down
11. muscle, fat
12. ten
13. amennorhea
14. muscles, one-third
15. water
16. cardiovascular, respiratory
17. moderate
18. fat
19. 48
20. a. rest
    b. carbohydrate
21. three
22. weight
23. carbohydrate, high
24. vitamin, mineral
25. fruit
26. liquid
27. four
28. energy
29. water
30. fatigue
31. 20,30
32. are not
33. magnesium, potassium
34. less
35. promote

36. iron
37. athlete's

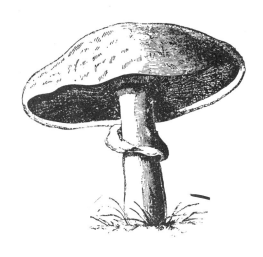

SELF TEST

1. Metabolism is the sum total of all the _____ reactions
    that go on in living cells.
    a. metabolic
    b. catabolic
    c. chemical
    d. anabolic

2. During digestion, carbohydrates are broken down to:
    a. monosaccharides and simple sugars.
    b. fructose and galactose.
    c. sucrose.
    d. glucoses.

3. Lipids are digested into basic units of:
    a. triglycerides.
    b. glycerol and fatty acids.
    c. mono-glycerides.

4. Protein is digested to:
    a. amino acids.
    b. lipoproteins.
    c. dipeptides.

5. When small molecules are put together to form larger ones,
    the reaction taking place is:
    a. anabolic.
    b. catabolic.
    c. alcoholic.
    d. none of the above.

6. When large molecules are broken down to smaller ones, the
    reaction taking place is:
    a. anabolic.
    b. catabolic.
    c. alchoholic.
    d. none of the above

7. Anabolic reactions involve:
    a. oxidation.
    b. reduction.
    c. both of the above

8. Catabolic reactions involve:
    a. oxidation.
    b. reduction.
    c. both of the above

9. Where does the body get its energy?
    a. from gluconeogensis
    b. from glycogenolysis
    c. from lipolysis
    d. from nutrients

10. The step from pyruvate to acetyl CoA is metabolically:
    a. reversible.
    b. irreversible.

11. The process by which acetyl CoA splits and releases its
    energy is known as the:
    a. TCA cycle.
    b. Krebs cycle.
    c. ATP cycle.
    d. Both a and b

12. Almost all dietary fats are:
    a. triglycerides.
    b. glycerol.
    c. cholesterol.
    d. none of the above

13. In a triglyceride that contains 54 carbon atoms, how many
    can become part of glucose?
    a. 3
    b. 9
    c. 43
    d. 54

14. If necessary for energy, what percentage of amino acids can
     be converted to provide glucose?
     a. 25%
     b. 50%
     c. 75%
     d. none
     e. 100%

15. Gluconeogenesis is a process in which:
     a. glucose is made from protein or fat.
     b. glucose is made from acetyl CoA.
     c. glucose is made from fatty acids.
     d. glucose is produced from the TCA Cycle.

16. Glycolysis is:
     a. the metabolic breakdown of glucose to pyruvate.
     b. the synthesis of acetyl CoA.
     c. reactions that convert glucose to glycogen.
     d. all of the above
     e. none of the above

17. When you remove nitrogen from protein, the process is
     called:
     a. determination.
     b. discrimination.
     c. deamination.
     d. nitrogination.

18. The principal nitrogen-excretion produce is called:
     a. nitrogination.
     b. sulfur.
     c. glycogen.
     d. urea.

19. Carbon-containing compounds that supply energy to the body
     are:
     a. carbohydrate, fat, protein, and alcohol.
     b. carbohydrate, fat, protein.
     c. carbohydrate, fat, protein and vitamins.
     d. protein and vitamins.
     e. all of the above

20. A food has the following composition: water, 50 grams;
     protein, 25 grams; carbohydrate, 10 grams; and fat, 10
     grams. A serving of the food contains:
     a. 200.
     b. 230.
     c. 440.
     d. 330.

21. Metabolism favors _____ when you eat too
     much of any energy nutrients.
     a. homeostasis
     b. fat formation
     c. additional energy
     d. all of the above

22. All substances that go through the Krebs Cycle must first
     be converted to:
     a. glucoses.
     b. acetyl CoA.
     c. pyruvic acid.
     d. lactic acid.

23. As fasting continues, the body adapts by producing an
     alternate energy source:
     a. ketones.
     b. glycogen.
     c. proteingenesis.
     d. urea.

24. When a person is starving or fasting, the first use of
     protein will be:
     a. replacement of worn-out cells.
     b. rebuilding of tissues.
     c. to provide energy.
     d. all of the above.

25. During fasting, _____ fat is lost than being on a
     low-calorie diet.
     a. less
     b. more
     c. the same
     d. none of the above

26. Acetone breath indicates the following:
     a. dental problems.
     b. constipation.
     c. ketosis.
     d. alkalosis.

27. If Mary drank one Cola per day in addition to the amount of
     kcalories necessary to maintain her weight, how much weight
     would she gain in one year? (200 calories per bottle)
     a. 7 pounds
     b. 21 pounds
     c. 13 pounds
     d. 31 pounds

28. Which of the following activities is not part of basal metabolism?
    a. glandular activity
    b. respiration
    c. circulation of the blood
    d. digestion
    e. maintenance of body temperature

29. A by-product of energy expenditure is:
    a. feces.
    b. heat.
    c. carbon dioxide.
    d. fiber.
    e. all of the above

30. An athlete uses _____ more protein than an average person.
    a. no
    b. 10%
    c. 50%
    d. 25%

31. The best choice for an athlete who needs to rehydrate is:
    a. Gatorade.
    b. cool water.
    c. sweat replacer.
    d. diluted juice.
    e. b and c

32. Athletes can safely add muscle tissue by:
    a. taking protein supplements.
    b. following a high-protein diet.
    c. putting a demand on muscles, making them work harder.

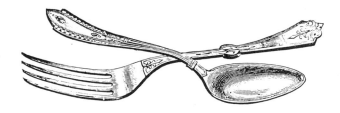

ANSWERS

1. c
2. a
3. b
4. a
5. a
6. b
7. b
8. a
9. d
10. b
11. e
12. a
13. a
14. b
15. b
16. a
17. c
18. d
19. a
20. b
21. b
22. b
23. a
24. c
25. a
26. c
27. b
28. d
29. b
30. b
31. e
32. c

EGGS, GOOD FOOD AT LOW COST...

Most people can eat 4-7 eggs a week without fear of raising their blood cholesterol levels. They are low in kcalories, rich in high-quality protein and a good source of iron and other minerals.

"FLIPPED" SMALL OMELET

Break 1 or 2 eggs into a small bowl. Mix briskly with a fork until all one color. Heat a pat of butter or margarine in a small skillet. When butter is melted and bubbly, pour egg mixture in. Take a fork and claw up the edges towards the center to build height and let uncooked portion run to outside. In a minute or two omelet will be ready to flip with a spatula. Heat in pan will finish cooking top, so take it off the burner. Immediately add cheese or other desired filling and fold in half and serve.

Miscellaneous tips

Since omelets cook very rapidly, have everything ready before you start, including the filling. Either make individual one- or two-egg omelets, or divide a larger one and provide seconds.

Although recipes vary, it is usually easier not to add either liquids or salt to the egg mixture before cooking the small, quick omelets.

If you mix diced cooked vegetables, chopped meat, etc. with the eggs before making the omelet, you have made an Italian "Frittata." Sometimes you can combine the French and Italian versions by using your imagination--such as mixing ham tidbits with the eggs and then using cheese for the filling. The fun part is using your imagination to produce a dish exactly to your own taste!

HARD-COOKED EGGS (not boiled!)

Can easily be made by starting in cold water, bringing
to a boil and gently simmering for about 15 minutes.
Alternate method is removing pan from heat entirely after
bringing eggs and water to a boil and covering pan tightly.
Let set about 20 minutes, plunge in cold water for easy peeling.

CHAPTER 7

Overweight and Underweight

YOU WILL LEARN . . .

1. The definition of obesity.

2. How many kcalories are in a pound of body fat.

3. How to determine ideal weight.

4. The difference between juvenile-onset obesity and adult-onset obesity.

5. The hazards of and causes of obesity.

6. What really is known about hunger and appetite, and the external and internal cues that signal eating behavior.

7. How obesity is unwisely treated and how it should be treated.

8. How to plan a weight loss diet that works.

9. The relationships between exercise and weight loss.

10. How to use behavior modification in a weight-control program.

11. The problems of underweight.

12. The definition of an eating disorder called anorexia nervosa.

HIGHLIGHT 7: SUGAR ADDICTION

13. Why we like sugar and why we can seem to be addicted to it.

14. How sugar has assumed an importance in some people's lives that it doesn't deserve.

15.   How we can cope with sugar without its harming us.

16.   New terms to understand: Sugar's "psychological effects," its "postingestive effect," and its action as a "supernormal immediate reinforcer."

CHAPTER 7: OVERWEIGHT AND UNDERWEIGHT

WEIGHT CONTROL

1. If you are too fat you are _____. If you are much too fat you are _____.

2. Energy itself doesn't weigh anything but when it exists in the form of _____ _____ in nutrients or body fat, the material that it holds together is both heavy and _____.

3. A pound of body fat stores _____ kcal.

IDEAL WEIGHT AND BODY FATNESS

4. Body weight says nothing about body _____.

5. Fat probably should make up about _____ percent of a man's body weight and about _____ percent of a woman's.

6. Ways of measuring fatness include:
   a. Weighing under water.
   b. Injecting a water-soluble substance into the lean tissue.
   c. The fatfold test (or skinfold test).
   d. The mirror test.
   e. Use of the _____ and height and weight tables. This involves a lot of guesswork.

7. a. A person more than _____ percent above ideal weight is considered overweight.
   b. Overweight by 15-20 percent or more is considered _____.
   c. Body weight more than _____ percent below normal is considered underweight.

CHAPTER 7: OVERWEIGHT AND UNDERWEIGHT

THE PROBLEM OF OBESITY

8. In the United States some 10-15 percent of all teenagers and some _____ to _____ percent of all adults are _____.

9. Obesity arising after adolescence is called reactive obesity or _____ - _____ obesity.

10. Obesity arising in childhood is called developmental obesity or _____ - _____ obesity.

11. Early overfeeding is thought to increase the _____ of fat cells.

12. Critical periods in life when body fat increases more rapidly than lean tissue are: early infancy, preadolescence, and the last three months of _____.

Hazards of Obesity

13. Insurance companies report that fat people die younger from heart attacks, strokes, diabetes, high blood pressure, complications from surgery, female problems, arthritis, gout, accidents, and the toxemia of _____.

14. Some fad diets are more _____ to health than obesity itself.

15. Besides physical disadvantages, there are also _____ and _____ disadvantages for the fat person.

16. Obesity is _____ (reversible/irreversible).

17. Many risks of obesity are _____ (reversible/irreversible).

CAUSES OF OBESITY

18. Obesity results from _____.

19. The problem of why people overeat _____ (has/has not) been solved.

20. Different points of view include: The set-point theory, environment, heredity. _____ (All/none) of them may be involved.

21. Families that allow their children to skip meals may be
    _____ (promoting/preventing) obesity.

Hunger and Appetite Regulation

22. Hunger is _____, an inborn instinct.

23. Appetite is _____, a learned response to food.

24. Satiety signals that it is time to _____ eating.

25. The glucostatic theory of hunger proposes that the
    _____ _____ level determines hunger.

26. The thermostatic theory suggests that the _____ of our
    _____ regulates our body weight.

27. The lipostatic theory states that the size of our
    _____ stores affect hunger.

28. The purinergic theory proposes that it is the circulating
    levels of _____, molecules found in _____ and
    _____ that regulate our eating behavior.

29. The brain area that seems to regulate aspects of eating
    behavior is the _____.

The Behavior of Eating

30. The substitution of one behavior for another under stress
    is called _____ _____.

31. Events that cause stress (stressors) and "_____
    _____" also affect eating behavior.

External Cues

32. Rather than waiting for hunger to signal a need to eat,
    some people with a weight problem eat at certain times of
    the day, because food is available, or because it looks or
    _____ good.

33. Some experiments show that _____ people have an
    internal "kcalorie counter" that seems to adjust their
    kcalorie intake while _____ people respond more to
    habit and other external factors.

CHAPTER 7: OVERWEIGHT AND UNDERWEIGHT

Stressors and Arousal

Note: The term "arousal" used here means increased activity of certain brain centers associated with excitement and anxiety.

34.   "Stressors" include pain, anxiety, arousal, excitement, and even the presence of _____.

35.   The brain produces endogenous _____ to soothe pain and lessen arousal. This enhances appetite for palatable foods, reduces activity, and helps explain why some people can gain weight in response to _____ while other people lose it.

36.   Hunger and appetite are connected to deep _____ needs and complex human sensations such as yearning, _____, addiction, or compulsion.

37.   Another problem is that food is used for non-nutritive purposes such as a substitute for _____ or friendship, to ward off _____ or relieve _____. Some eating might be just for entertainment!

38.   Stress prepares the body for physical action, and the same mechanism operates during emotional stress. Thus, released glucose is transferred into fat and the lowered glucose level signals _____. What a cycle to be in!

39.   Stress eating appears in many different _____.

Inactivity

40.   The most important single contributor to obesity in our country is _____.

41.   The control of hunger/appetite works quite well in active people but _____ when activity falls below a certain level.

42.   Obese people are usually extremely _____.

Individuality

43.   No two people are alike, either physically or _____.

44.   The top priority should be _____ of obesity.

CHAPTER 7: OVERWEIGHT AND UNDERWEIGHT

TREATMENTS OF OBESITY: POOR CHOICES
Water Pills

45. An overfat person has a smaller percentage of body water and dehydrating oneself does nothing to solve the _____ problem.

Diet Pills, Starch Blockers, and Glucomannan

46. How many drugs are both safe and effective for the treatment of obesity? _____

47. Diet pills, which are widely used _____ (are/are not) safe.

48. Starch blockers _____ (have/have not) helped people lose weight.

49. A preparation derived from a Japanese vegetable (konjac tuber) is called _____. Controlled tests have found it _____ (effective/ineffective) in weight control.

50. Two promising candidates for the future may be _____ and _____ _____.

Health Spas

51. Health spa machines and baths _____ (do/do not) offer real advantage for weight control.

52. The idea of there being two kinds of fat, one called _____, has turned out to be a money-making _____.

53. The author of a book that published misinformation cannot be sued unless a customer can prove that the book has caused _____ _____.

54. Most books available to the public about nutrition contain _____.

55. The most reliable publications about nutrition information are the _____ _____.

Hormones

56. It has been hoped for a long time that a _____ might be found that would promote weight _____.

57. Thyroid hormone causes loss of _____ _____ mass and _____ problems.

58. HCG has proved _____ (effective/ineffective) and weight loss with HCG has occurred only because of a _____ kcal diet.

Surgery

59. Bypass surgery is a relatively safe procedure designed to help patients absorb less of what they eat. There are no side effects.   a. True   b. False

Fad diets

60. Fad diets _____ (are/are not) recommended in the treatment of obesity.

THE SUCCESSFUL TREATMENT OF OBESITY

61. Only one-third of the people succeed in keeping weight off after reducing. Their success is the result of a combination of diet, exercise, and _____ _____.

Diet

Diet comes from the Greek word <u>diata</u> which means "way of life". A diet is not something to go on and off, but the way one eats for the rest of his or her life.

62. The key is adopting an "_____ _____" rather than a "diet."

63. In planning a regular weight <u>maintenance</u> diet, the following balance is suggested:
    a. _____ percent of kcal from protein.
    b. _____ percent of kcal (or less) from fat.
    c. _____ percent of kcal or more from carbohydrate.

64. For weight loss, cut the fat grams in half, leave the
    protein as is and get the rest from carbohydrate.
    Translated into grams on a 1200 kcalories diet, this would
    be:
    a. _____ grams protein, or _____ kcal.
    b. _____ grams fat, or _____ kcal.
    c. _____ grams CHO, or _____ kcal.

65. It is important to adopt a _____ plan, because
    you will be staying with it for the rest of your life.
    Most people just can't get this concept that your everyday
    eating plan is what counts, not the two-week, four-week or
    six-week "wonder diet" that entraps gullible people who
    believe in magic rather than facts.

66. A helpful attitude to adopt is "I _____ myself, and I'm
    going to take _____ _____ of me"

67. Take a _____ view of yourself.

68. _____ weighs more than oxidized fat, so sometimes,
    during weight-loss, one will appear not to lose weight, or
    to even gain weight temporarily. It is important to
    understand this to avoid becoming discouraged.

69. It is easier to _____ a food than to _____ away
    its kcalories.

Exercise

70. No exercise enables you to _____ reduce.

71. You can change your body shape only by changing your
    posture and _____ structure.

Behavior Modification

72. If you want to lose weight, learn to eat more _____.
    If you want to gain weight, eat more food within the first
    _____ minutes of a meal.

73. Sensible suggestions that can work include:
    a. including soup in meals.
    b. joining Weight Watchers, TOPS, or other reliable
       self-help groups.
    c. keeping a record of circumstances that trigger
       eating.
    d. assertiveness training.
    e. not cleaning your _____.

The Problem of Underweight

74. Causes of death seen more often in thin people, but not
     entirely related to underweight, are tuberculosis, cancer
     and _____ .

75. Underweight can be caused by psychological factors,
     metabolic differences, and a _____ component. In
     addition, thin people are very often extremely active.

Note: One wise person once said, "A fat person lives to eat,
       a thin one eats to live."

76. Strategies recommended for weight gain include making
     high-kcalorie choices of nutritious foods, eating liberal
     servings, and regularly _____ between meals.

Anorexia Nervosa

Note: The term anorexia means loss of appetite and this can be
a complication of the flu or other bodily disorders. Anorexia
nervosa, meaning "nervous loss of appetite," is a medical term
used to refer to "the starving disease" described in the text.
Now that more is known about this disorder, we find it was
poorly named. Those suffering from anorexia nervosa do have an
appetite and spend much time thinking about food or even
preparing it for others. If the condition persists for some
time, however, the body's digestive system suffers from abuse to
the point where normal eating becomes almost impossible for the
victim. It is actually ferocious control over appetite rather
than lack of appetite that describes this condition more
exactly.

SUMMING UP

Review Test

Check with your instructor to see if there is a diet planning
self-study assignment. If not, you may still want to do this
exercise on your own.

CHAPTER 7:   ANSWERS

1.   overweight, obese
2.   chemical bonds, visible
3.   3,500
4.   composition
5.   18, 22
6.   scales
7.   a. 10, b. obese, c. 10
8.   25, 50, obese
9.   adult-onset
10.   juvenile-onset
11.   number
12.   pregnancy
13.   pregnancy
14.   hazardous
15.   social, economic
16.   reversible
17.   reversible
18.   overeating
19.   has not
20.   all
21.   promoting
22.   physiological
23.   psychological
24.   stop
25.   blood glucose
26.   rate, metabolism
27.   fat
28.   purines, DNA, RNA
29.   hypothalamus
30.   displacement activity
31.   external cues
32.   tastes
33.   thin, fat
34.   food
35.   opiates, stress
36.   emotional, craving

37. love, depression, boredom
38. hunger
39. patterns
40. underactivity
41. fails
42. inactive
43. psychologically
44. prevention
45. fat
46. none
47. are not
48. have not
49. glucomannan, ineffective
50. naloxone, sucrose polyester
51. do not
52. cellulite, hoax
53. bodily harm
54. misinformation
55. scientific journals
56. hormone, loss
57. lean body, heart
58. ineffective, low
59. b. F
60. are not
61. behavior modification
62. eating plan
63. a. 15, b. 30, c. 55
64. a. 90, 360
     b. 40, 360
     c. 120, 480
65. realistic
66. like, good care
67. positive
68. Water
69. exclude, exercise
70. spot
71. muscle
72. slowly, 20
73. plate
74. suicide
75. genetic
76. snacking

HIGHLIGHT 7: SUGAR ADDICTION

1. We all have a _____ and _____ relationship with our food.

The Sweet Taste

2. The reward of sweetness makes sugar an _____ _____.   Since the pleasure is so intense, sugar is known as a _____ immediate reinforcer.

3. If our appetite has been satisfied by eating sugar, another reinforcer, the _____ _____ is in operation.

4. Addictive drugs such as _____ are also supernormal, positive reinforcers.

5. It is important not to eat sugar's empty kcalories when your body's need is for _____ _____.

6. Some people turn to sugar so often it seems like a truly _____ _____.

The Case for Sugar as an Addictive Drug

7. A person addicted to sugar could be called a "sugarholic, " _____," or "_____."

8. A more accurate description than addiction is sugar _____.

9. Rat experiments showed a relationship between a low-_____ diet and excessive reliance on sugar.

10. Sugar contributes to malnutrition (directly/indirectly) _____.

HIGHLIGHT 7: SUGAR ADDICTION

Sugar Eating and Puritanism

11. The puritanical attitude makes every meal become an
     experience in which an individual must decide between doing
     _____ or _____ himself.

12. Sugar is seen as _____ - _____ by those who hate
     and fear it.

13. Binge eating is called _____ or _____.

14. Binge eaters are especially controlled by the powerful
     emotional attraction of _____.

How Can We Cope with Sugar?

15. Sugar is a harmless and _____ substance.

16. Children live for the _____. _____ protect their
     _____.

17. Everyone should _____ to eat the foods they need
     first.

ANSWERS

1.   complex, intense
2.   immediate reinforcer, supernormal
3.   postingestive effect
4.   opiates
5.   nutritious food
6.   addictive substance
7.   carboholic, sucroholic
8.   abuse
9.   protein
10. indirectly
11. right, enjoying
12. all-powerful
13. bulimia, bulimarexia
14. sugar
15. unneeded
16. present. You, future
17. learn

CHAPTER 7: OVERWEIGHT AND UNDERWEIGHT

SELF TEST

1. A person weighing 170 pounds, whose ideal weight is 150 pounds, is:
   a. overweight.
   b. obese.
   c. chunky.
   d. pudgy
   e. at risk for thyroid problems.

2. - 5. Matching. Match the eating vocabulary word with the correct definition.
   a. The physiological need to eat.
   b. The psychological desire to eat.
   c. Something that stimulates eating such as the smell or taste of food.
   d. a feeling of fullness or satisfaction after a meal.

2. _____ satiety

3. _____ hunger

4. _____ appetite

5. _____ external cue

6. The cells of an obese person become less responsive to his hormone, causing excessive production of the hormone.
   a. insulin
   b. cholecystokinin
   c. gastrin
   d. thyroxine

CHAPTER 7: OVERWEIGHT AND UNDERWEIGHT

7. Protein should not be cut too low on a sensible weight loss diet because:
   a. It adds satiety value to a meal.
   b. It aids in burning up fat.
   c. It cannot be converted to fat.
   d. It has fewer kcalories per gram than carbohydrate.
   e. all of the above

8. **For** nutrition adequacy, it is wise to consume a diet **that** contains at least:
   a. 200 kcalories.
   b. 1800 kcalories.
   c. 1200 kcalories.
   d. 700 kcalories a day.
   e. 500 kcalories.

9. Feelings of fullness from a meal are sent to the brain after a _____ lag.
   a. 5 minute
   b. 10 minute
   c. 20 minute
   d. 45 minute

10. Which of the following nutrients can supply energy to the body?
    a. Water
    b. Vitamins
    c. Minerals
    d. all of the above
    e. none of the above

11. Obesity can be completely explained by:
    a. the glucostatic theory.
    b. the thermostatic theory.
    c. the lipostatic theory.
    d. all of the above
    e. none of the above

12. If you eat 2400 kcalories a day, about _____ will be used up for the "specific dynamic effect" of food.
    a. 24 kaclories
    b. 240 kcalories
    c. 100 kcalories
    d. 10 kcalories
    e. 3500 kcalories

13. There is no Recommended Dietary Allowance (RDA) for:
     a. Protein.
     b. Carbohydrate.
     c. Energy.
     d. all of the above

14. Which of the following activities is <u>not</u> included in the
     measurement of BMR?
     a. Energy cost of the heart beating
     b. Energy cost of digesting food
     c. Energy cost of maintaining your body temperature
     d. Energy cost of the lungs operating

15. One of the byproducts of oxidizing body fat is water.
     a. true
     b. false

16. An example of a behavior modification technique for weight
     control is:
     a. Feel guilty after you overeat.
     b. Have someone nag you if you overeat.
     c. Keep a record of your eating habits so you can see what
         situations cause you to overeat.

17. A lack of appetite is know as anorexia.
     a. true
     b. false

18. Weight losses on a low carbohydrate diet are due to:
     a. Nausea and appetite restriction due to ketosis.
     b. Reduction of kcalorie intake due to the difficulty of
         planning a palatable low carbohydrate diet.
     c. High levels of water loss in the urine.
     d. all of the above

19. Usually a low carbohydrate diet allows no more than:
     a. 5 grams of carbohydrate per day.
     b. 15 grams
     c. 60 grams
     d. 110 grams
     e. 300 grams

20. Obesity that arises early in life is called:
     a. Adult-onset obesity.
     b. Maturity-onset obesity.
     c. Developmental obesity.
     d. Early-onset obesity.
     e. none of the above

21. Obesity that arises later in life is called:
    a. Adult-onset obesity.
    b. Maturity-onset obesity.
    c. Developmental obesity.
    d. Early-onset obesity.
    e. none of the above

22. Underweight is associated with an increased risk of:
    a. Heart attack.
    b. Kidney failure.
    c. Infection.
    d. None of the above

23. Fat loss is enhanced by:
    a. Regular exercise.
    b. Behavior modification.
    c. both of the above
    d. None of the above

24. Mortality risk in obesity is:
    a. Irreversible.
    b. Reversible.
    c. Linear.
    d. All of the above

25. One of the oldest and most popular reducing diets is the:
    a. Low-carbohydrate diet.
    b. Low-protein diet.
    c. High-fat diet.
    d. Low-fat diet.

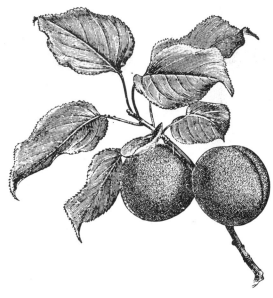

ANSWERS

1.   b
2.   d
3.   a
4.   b
5.   c
6.   a
7.   a
8.   c
9.   c
10.   e
11.   e
12.   b
13.   b
14.   b
15.   a
16.   c
17.   a
18.   d
19.   c
20.   c
21.   a
22.   c
23.   c
24.   b
25.   a

RECIPES YOU CAN TRY...

There are excellent books on the market devoted to low-kcalorie cookery. Exercise and persistence in following a healthy way of life will pay off.

The following recipes are included to provide some ideas to get you started. They feature vegetables, and are wise choices for high nutrient density, and limited kcalories. One of the most important things to remember in controlling weight is to eat a balanced diet and remember that a "diet" is a way of life, not something to go on and off of periodically.

MARINATED VEGETABLES

1 large green pepper, cut into 1/2-inch pieces
1 large sweet red pepper, cut into thin 2-inch-long strips
4 carrots, sliced diagonally into 1/4-inch pieces

1/2 pound fresh mushrooms, sliced lengthwise (or left whole if very small)
1-2 small red onions, finely chopped or 3-4 green onions finely chopped
1/2 cup Vinaigrette Dressing (recipe follows)

Mix all ingredients together well. Cover and chill for 1 or 2 hours before serving.

Size of Serving: 1 cup
Number of Servings: 8, 35 kcalories per serving.
Excellent Source of: Vitamin A, Riboflavin, and Vitamin C

VINAIGRETTE DRESSING

3 tbsp vegetable oil
5 tbsp wine vinegar
2 tbsp fresh lemon juice

2 tbsp finely minced shallots or green onions

6 tbsp water
1 tsp Dijon-style
   mustard
1 large garlic clove,
   crushed

1 tbsp honey
1 tsp crushed tarragon
1/4 tsp paprika
1/8 tsp freshly ground
   pepper
Salt to taste (optional)

Mix well in a tightly covered jar; store in refrigerator.

Yield: 1 cup, 30 kcalories per tbsp

GAZPACHO BY THE CUPFUL

1 medium tomato, peeled
   and diced
1/4 cucumber, peeled and
   chopped

1 tbsp chopped onion
2 sprigs parsley, chopped
1/8 tsp garlic powder
Dash hot pepper sauce

Combine all ingredients in blender and liquify.
Chill and serve.

Size of Serving: 1 cup, 50 kcalories.
Excellent Source of: Iron, Vitamin A, and Vitamin C

SAUTEED FRESH VEGETABLES WITH SEASONED YOGURT

This blend of fresh vegetable flavors goes with any main
dish or serve it as a main dish with whole-grain bread.
Delicious hot or cold.

1 eggplant, diced
1/4 cup vegetable oil
1 onion, sliced
2 green peppers, slices
1 zucchini, cut in strips
1 crookneck summer
   squash (yellow)
   sliced lengthwise
2 tomatoes, quartered

1 cup thickly sliced large
   fresh mushrooms
Fresh basil (if available)
1/4 cup fresh parsley
Salt to taste
Ground black pepper
   to taste
1 cup plain lowfat yogurt
1 clove garlic, crushed

Salt the eggplant let it drain for 1/2 hour, then squeeze
and dry slices.

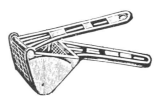

CHAPTER 8

The Water-Soluble Vitamins: B Vitamins and Vitamin C

YOU WILL LEARN

1. Which vitamins are classified as water soluble.

2. What the general characteristics of the B-vitamins are, their functions, and which foods they are found in.

3. The role of B-vitamins in the glucose-to-energy pathway.

4. How prescription drugs interfere with action of the B-vitamins.

5. Common symptoms of a B-vitamin deficiency.

6. What foods contain B-vitamins, and how much of each separate vitamin is considered adequate for normal people.

7. More about "non-B" vitamins.

8. The metabolic roles of vitamin C.

9. Signs of vitamin C deficiencies and the recommended intakes.

10. The facts about vitamin C toxicity.

11. What to eat that supplies vitamin C.

HIGHLIGHT 8A: ALCOHOL AND NUTRITION

12. What happens to alcohol in the body.

13. How alcohol affects the user.

14. How to drink socially and what helps (and doesn't help) to sober someone up.

15.   The types of malnutrition resulting from alcohol use.

HIGHLIGHT 8B: RUMORS VERSUS RESEARCH

16.   The problem of designing an experiment that truly tests whether or not a nutrient is effective in helping symptoms or curing a disease.

17.   The difference between experiments depending on whether the researcher as well as the experimental groups knows who is receiving the specified treatment.

18.   How difficult it is to reach conclusions about scientific studies unless you know how the experiment was conducted and the sample size.

19.   What "replication" of an experiment means.

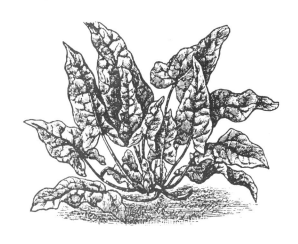

The Water-Soluble Vitamins: B and C

WATER-SOLUBLE VITAMINS

1. B-vitamins come together in _____, they work together in
    the _____. Think of them as a team!

2. Water-soluble vitamins travel easily in the
    _____.

3. Water-soluble vitamins are less likely to be _____ in
    the body, but they are very easily _____.

4. Vitamin B-2, riboflavin, is easy to see when excesses are
    excreted. It turns your _____ a bright yellow.

5. In summary, the water-soluble vitamins are:
    a. carried in the bloodstream
    b. excreted in urine
    c. unlikely to be toxic
    d. needed in _____ _____ doses

Coenzymes

6. A coenzyme is a small _____molecule that associates
    closely with an _____.

7. If a coenzyme is part of the enzyme structure, it is known
    as a _____ group.

8. Others participate in the reaction being performed and are
    _____ altered in the process, but are always
    _____ sooner or later.

9. Still other coenzymes are unaltered but form part of
    the_____site of the enzyme. The active site is
    where the reaction takes place.

10. Thiamin, Vitamin B-1, is involved in glucose catabolism in the breakdown of pyruvate to _____ _____.

11. The breakdown of glucose to pyruvate utilizes Vitamin B-3, or _____.

12. Breaking down acetyl CoA to carbon dioxide involves _____ _____.

13. The glucose-to-_____ pathway would not function without thiamin, riboflavin, niacin and pantothenic acid.

14. Symptoms of niacin deficiency include major breakdowns in the body known as the "four Ds":
    a. _____ b. _____
    c. _____ d. _____

15. The complete breakdown of amino acids and _____ depend on the same coenzymes.

16. Anabolism (building) and catabolism (breakdown) of compounds depend on coenzymes. Transamination of protein is associated with vitamin _____, pyridoxine.

17. _____(and B_{12}cobalamin) are involved in cell division and reproduction of the genetic code, DNA and RNA.

18. _____ is a coenzyme involved in fat synthesis.

B VITAMINS AND PRESCRIPTION DRUGS

19. Prescription drugs often interfere with the action of the B vitamins:

    a. A tuberculosis drug, INH, is a vitamin _____ antagonist.
    b. Aspirin interferes with the absorption of _____ as well as vitamin C and iron.
    c. Alcohol and other drugs also interfere with nutrition.

B-VITAMIN DEFICIENCY

20. A B-vitamin deficiency seldom shows up in _____.

21. The thiamin-deficiency disease is called
     _____.
     The niacin-deficiency disease is called
     _____.
     But even in these cases the deficiencies are not
     _____.

22. It is really not natural to take any kind of _____ at
     all.

23. The skin and _____ appear to be especially
     sensitive to vitamin B deficiencies, but their
     abnormalities are only outward manifestations of what is
     happening inside the body.

24. A skin rash is a _____, not a disease.

THE B VITAMINS IN FOOD

25. The RDA for thiamin for adults is about _____ for men
     and about _____ for women. More is needed when energy
     expenditure is _____.

26. You need just as much _____ when you are fasting as at
     any other time because it is related to energy expenditure.

27. The RDA for riboflavin is about 1.4 to _____ mg. for men
     and about 1.1 to _____ mg. for women.

Riboflavin

28. The major contributors of riboflavin among the food groups
     are _____ and _____.

29. Riboflavin can be destroyed by the light from sun or
     _____ lamps.

Niacin

30. Niacin can be obtained from another source, _____.

31. The amino acid _____ can be converted to
     _____ in the body at the ratio of _____ mg of
     tryptophan yielding _____ of niacin.

32. Tryptophan is also needed to build needed body proteins so
     not all of it is available for making _____.

191

33. Vegetarians are advised to emphasize _____ and
    _____ in their diets as good sources of niacin and
    _____.

34. Insanity caused by a lack of niacin has symptoms similar to
    those of _____.

35. A branch of psychiatry that attempts to treat mental
    illness by correcting nutrient imbalances and deficiencies
    is called _____psychiatry.

36. Large doses of niacin seem to lower blood _____
    but niacin causes irritation of the _____ and
    possible liver damage.

37. An alternative form of niacin, called _____
    seems ineffective in treating cholesterol problems.

38. A niacin _____ results from a megadose as well as a
    stinging sensation that is sometimes painful.

Vitamin B$_6$

39. Two mg of vitamin B$_6$ per day is enough to handle
    100 g of _____. This coenzyme is very
    important in _____ _____ metabolism.

40. Pregnant women need about _____ a milligram more due to
    the high demand for vitamin B$_6$ by the fetus. More
    may also be needed by women taking oral _____.

41. The richest food sources seem to be muscle meats, liver,
    vegetables, and _____-_____cereals.

Folacin

42. The U.S. RDA for folacin is _____ micrograms a day
    with _____ micrograms added for pregnancy.

Note: you can remember the name "folacin" easily if you relate
it to the word "foliage". Dark-green leafy vegetables are a
wonderful source as well as many fruits and vegetables.

43. Folacin is easily destroyed by cooking. Salad greens and
    _____ fruits are dependable sources.

44. Folacin deficiency affects all rapidly dividing cells
(because of making new DNA and RNA). Especially affected
are the _____ tract, the body's _____-_____
sites, and transport and absorption of other nutrients and
oxygen.

45. Folacin deficiency depresses _____.

46. Folacin deficiency also affects the _____, nervous
system, and behavior. Fatigue, depression, confusion, poor
memory, and disorientation can result as well.

47. Folacin deficiencies may result from inadequate intake,
impaired _____, or _____ metabolic need.
Deficiencies from all three causes are _____.

48. An inadequate intake is seen in babies fed _____ milk.
Overconsumers of _____ or empty-kcalorie items are
vulnerable. Many of the neurological _____ seen in
alcoholism are caused by _____ deficiency.

49. Deficiencies can also be caused by having greater needs
such as multiple pregnancy, _____, chicken pox,
measles, burns, etc.

50. Risks of overdosing with folacin are _____ than
those for the other B vitamins discussed so far.

Vitamin B$_{12}$

51. Only _____ micrograms of B$_{12}$ is needed by the
adult. This can also be written _____mg.

52. It is found only in _____ _____ such as meat,
milk, cheese, and eggs. Strict vegetarians must take
supplements or use fortified soy milk.

53. Another special characteristic is that it requires an
"_____ _____," a
mucopolysaccharide made in the stomach, for absorption.

54. The disorder caused by lack of intrinsic factor is called
_____ anemia and it causes a creeping paralysis of
the nerves and muscles as well as immature red blood cells.

55. _____ will normalize the blood cells, but not
the creeping paralysis.

CHAPTER 8: THE WATER-SOLUBLE VITAMINS

56. It may actually take _____ for a deficiency to develop in a new vegetarian, giving him or her a false sense of security.

57. The breast-fed infant of a _____ mother may be the first to suffer.

58. At one time, people who had pernicious anemia had to eat several pounds of _____ a day in order to survive.

59. The word "intrinsic" means inside or part of and _____ means outside the system, or separate.

Pantothenic Acid and Biotin

60. Pantothenic acid and _____ are needed for the _____ of coenzymes. They are both _____ (hard to find/easy to find) in foods.

61. _____ deficiencies would probably be found only if artificial feedings were used that lacked _____, and if antibiotics killed intestinal bacteria.

62. Large amounts of raw _____ whites produce a deficiency in _____.

63. The only other problem with biotin involves _____ disorders.

Non-B Vitamins

64. Three compounds serve as coenzymes in metabolism, but are very abundantly found in foods. They are _____, _____ and _____ acid.

65. Findings in certain articles and claims were based on _____ studies and haven't been applicable to _____ beings.

66. When a normal dose of a nutrient clears up a deficiency it is having a _____ effect. When a megadose overwhelms some system and acts like a drug, the nutrient is having a _____ effect. (Note the relationship of this word to "pharmacy").

67. Choline and related lecithins, used as drugs instead of as nutrients, have been beneficial in Alzheimer's disease and _____ dyskinesia.

68. A rule of thumb in understanding use of certain substances
    might be that what is "bad" high may be "good" _____
    and that _____ is not necessarily better.

69. Other substances mistaken for essential nutrients include
    _____, _____, and ubiquinone.

VITAMIN C

70. The vitamin C deficiency disease is called
    _____.

71. The anti-scurvy substance in limes and citrus fruits became
    known as the _____ factor, now called
    _____ _____, a 6-carbon compound similar to
    _____.

72. There are two active forms of vitamin C, one is
    _____ acid. Any amount over _____mg is
    considered a _____.

Metabolic Roles of Vitamin C

73. In spite of all that is written and known about this
    substance, much is still not _____.

74. Vitamin C has to "be present" for certain _____ to
    occur but the exact _____ of its action is still being
    studied.

75. Some of its roles may be to act as a coenzyme, cofactor, or
    _____.

Collagen Formation

76. The best understood role of vitamin C is in
    _____ formation.

77. Vitamin C catches _____ ions and reconverts them to the
    _____ form so the enzyme can keep on working.

Antioxidant Action

78. Any substance that can donate electrons to another is a
    _____ agent; when it donates its electrons it
    reduces another compound and simultaneously becomes
    _____ itself.

79. Many substances found in food can be altered or even destroyed by _____.

80. Vitamin C can protect other substances by being _____ itself.

The Absorption of Iron

81. A molecule that can assume a form suitable for trapping ions with two positive charges like a magnetic pair of pliers is called a _____agent.

82. Eating foods containing vitamin C at the same meal with foods containing _____ can double or triple the absorption of _____from those foods.

83. Multicolored, mixed dishes probably please the body, the eye, and the _____ more than single foods.

Amino Acid Metabolism

84. Some amino acids end up being converted to hormones such as norepinephrine and _____.

85. Stress _____ the need for vitamin C.

86. Vitamin C is also involved in the fever _____ to infection.

87. Infections and exposure to _____ also increase your needs.

Vitamin C and Other Nutrients

88. Vitamin C may aid the body in using _____. It also interacts with _____.

VITAMIN C DEFICIENCY

89. Widespread deficiencies of vitamin C _____ (still/no longer) exist.

90. With an adequate intake, the body maintains a _____ _____ of vitamin C and rapidly _____ any excess in the _____.

91. The pool becomes depleted at the rate of about _____ percent a day when there is an inadequate intake.

92. Vitamin C shifts unpredictably between the _____ and the
     _____ blood cells known as _____ .

93. Two early signs of scurvy are _____ gums and
     _____ .

94. Sudden death in scurvy is caused by massive
     _____ .

95. Scurvy can be reversed in _____ days using _____mg per
     day of vitamin C.

RECOMMENDED INTAKES OF VITAMIN C

96. Recommendations for already healthy people vary from a low
     of _____ mg per day in Britain and Canada to
     _____ mg in Germany. The U.S. RDA is _____mg.

97. At an intake of _____mg. per day, 95% of the population
     probably reach a maximum pool size.

98. Among stresses known to increase vitamin C needs are
     infections, burns, high or low temperature, toxic levels of
     heavy metals, the chronic use of medications including
     aspirin, barbiturates, and oral _____ .

99. Cigarette _____ increases the vitamin C need to at
     least _____ mg. per day.

VITAMIN C. TOXICITY

100. Toxic effects can theoretically include formation of
      _____ in the kidneys, upset of the body's
      _____-_____ balance, destruction of vitamin _____ , and
      interference with the action of vitamin _____ .

101. Toxic effects of immediate concern involve _____ ,
      abdominal cramps, diarrhea, interference with medical
      _____ . Megadoses of vitamin C can make red blood
      cells _____ in persons with an inherited _____
      deficiency.

102. The emergence of withdrawal symptoms from drug overdose
      does not prove a _____ . If everyone truly
      followed the Basic 4 recommendation of four servings of
      fruits and vegetables, needs for vitamin C would be well
      met.

103.   Foods with excellent amounts of vitamin C besides citrus
       include broccoli, brussels sprouts, cantaloupe, and
       _____.

104.   The _____ determines vitamin C content of foods, so it
       is found mostly in _____ plants.

SUMMING UP

Review text if necessary.

Note the interesting projects suggested in the Self-Study
section of the text on the water-soluble vitamins.

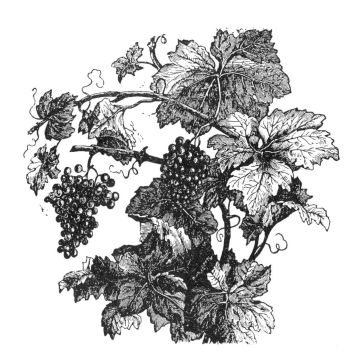

ANSWERS

1. foods, body
2. bloodstream
3. stored, destroyed
4. urine
5. frequent small
6. nonprotein, enzyme
7. prosthetic
8. chemically, regenerated
9. active
10. acetyl CoA
11. niacin
12. pantothenic acid
13. energy
14. a. dermatitis, b. dementia, c. diarrhea, d. death
15. fat
16. B_6
17. Folacin
18. Biotin
19. a. B_6 b. folacin
20. isolation
21. beriberi, pellagra, pure
22. pills
23. tongue
24. symptom
25. 1.5 mg, 1.0 mg, high.
26. thiamin
27. 1.7, 1.3
28. milk, meat
29. fluorescent
30. protein
31. tryptophan, niacin, 60, 1 mg
32. niacin
33. nuts, legumes, protein
34. schizophrenia
35. orthomolecular

36. cholesterol, intestines
37. niacinamide
38. flush
39. protein, amino acid
40. half, contraceptives
41. whole-grain
42. 400, 400.
43. citrus
44. GI, blood making
45. immunity
46. brain
47. absorption, unusual, common
48. goat's, alcohol, abnormalities, folacin
49. cancer
50. greater
51. 3, .003
52. animal products
53. intrinsic factor
54. pernicious
55. Folacin
56. years
57. vegan
58. liver
59. extrinsic
60   biotin, synthesis, easy to find
61. Biotin, biotin
62. egg, animals
63. genetic
64. inositol, choline, lipoic
65. animal, human
66. physiological, pharmacological
67. tardive
68. low, more
69. PABA, bioflavonoids
70. scurvy
71. antiscorbutic, ascorbic acid, glucose
72. ascorbic, 1000, megadose
73. understood
74. reactions, mechanism
75. antioxidant
76. collagen
77. ferric, ferrous
78. reducing, oxidized
79. oxidation
80. oxidized
81. chelating
82. iron, iron
83. palate
84. thyroxine

85. increases
86. response
87. cold
88. folacin, calcium
89. still
90. metabolic pool, excretes, urine
91. 3
92. plasma, white, leukocytes
93. bleeding, bruises
94. bleeding
95. five, 100
96. 30, 75, 60
97. 100
98. contraceptives
99. smoking, 140
100. stones, acid-base, B_{12}, E
101. nausea, regimes, burst, enzyme
102. need
103. strawberries,
104. sun, growing

HIGHLIGHT 8A   ALCOHOL AND NUTRITION

1. If liver cells could talk, they would describe alcohol as demanding, egocentric, and _____.

2. Liver cells prefer fatty acids as fuel, but when alcohol is present they are forced to use _____ and let the _____ _____ accumulate in huge stockpiles.

3. Alcohol affects every organ of the body, but the most dramatic evidence of its disruptive behavior appears in the _____.

4. Only _____ cells can get rid of alcohol.

Alcohol Enters the Body

5. To the chemist, _____ refers to a class of compounds containing reactive hydroxyl (OH) groups. The glycerol in triglycerides is an example of an _____ to a chemist.

6. To the average person, _____ refers to the intoxicating ingredient in beer or distilled spirits. The chemist's name for this particular alcohol is _____.

7. Ethanol has only _____ carbons and _____ hydroxyl group.

8. The name given the feeling of great well-being sought by humans through the use of drugs such as alcohol is called _____.

9. Absorption of alcohol can be slowed in the stomach if it is full of _____, especially _____ snacks or high-_____ foods.

Alcohol Arrives in the Liver

10. Each molecule of alcohol that enters the capillaries of the liver will tie up two molecules of _____ and one of _____ while being processed.

11. An overuser of alcohol is likely to be deficient in these two _____ .

12. Some racial groups have genetic information that makes them too uncomfortable when using alcohol to become _____ .

13. The enzyme that processes alcohol is called alcohol _____ .

14. Fasting _____(lowers/speeds up) the effect of alcohol.

15. If NADH keeps acetyl CoAs from getting into the TCA cycle where they are used for energy, they then become building blocks for _____ _____ .

16. An accumulation of uric acid crystals in the joints is called _____ .

17. Alcohol also slows amino acid _____ and weakens the _____ system.

18. Synthesis of lipoproteins speeds up, _____ (increasing/decreasing) blood triglyceride levels.

19. The first stage of liver deterioration in heavy drinkers is an accumulation of _____ . This interferes with the distribution of nutrients and _____ to the liver cells.

20. The second stage of liver deterioration is called _____ .

21. The last stage is called _____ and it is _____ (reversible/irreversible.)

22. The system that metabolizes both alcohol and drugs is called the MEOS, _____ ethanol oxidizing system.

23. The MEOS _____ (enlarges/shrinks) with repeated exposure to alcohol.

24. If the MEOS _____, it makes the body able to metabolize drugs much _____ than before.

Ethanol Arrives in the Brain

25. Alcohol continues to be used as a _____.

26. Alcohol is a depressant, not a _____.

27. The way that persons are affected by alcohol that is not processed is:
    a. interference with reasoning and _____ .
    b. speech and vision become _____.
    c. The area that governs reasoning becomes more incapacitated.
    d. motor control of large muscles deteriorates.
    e. The person "_____ _____."
    f. If he or she were able to continue drinking, the breathing and heartbeat would _____.

28. Liver cells and _____ cells die with exposure to _____. Brain cells _____(do/do not) regenerate.

29. The thirst caused by loss of body water can only be relieved by drinking _____.

30. In addition to water loss, important _____ are lost. Magnesium and _____ need to be normalized.

Drinking and Drunkenness

31. It takes about _____ hours to metabolize one drink. You should drink _____ with food and not _____ your drinks.

32. More muscle action _____ (will/will not) help metabolize alcohol.

33. Coffee _____ (will/will not) help metabolize alcohol.

34. 90% of the alcohol is cleared by the _____, 10% is excreted through the _____ and _____.

35. The amount of alcohol in the breath is in proportion to that still in the _____.

36. Legal drunkenness is defined by blood alcohol content of .10 to _____ percent.

37. It takes _____ hours for a body to clear alcohol completely.

38. Alcohol can damage the unborn baby's central _____ system as well as causing a deprivation of oxygen.

Drinking and Malnutrition

39. Alcohol can contribute to malnutrition in the following ways:
     a. Lack of _____. Too many kcalories from _____ instead of food.
     b. _____-vitamin depletion.

40. Well-nourished alcoholics can also suffer from _____ and folacin deficiency and _____ depletion.

41. Ethanol can also cause _____ and interfere with many chemical and hormonal reactions in the body.

ANSWERS

1. disruptive
2. alcohol, fatty acids
3. liver
4. liver
5. alcohol, alcohol
6. alcohol, ethanol
7. two, one
8. euphoria
9. food, carboydrate, fat
10. niacin, thiamin
11. vitamins
12. addicted
13. dehydrogenase
14. speeds up
15. fatty acids
16. gout
17. metabolism, immune
18. increasing
19. fat. oxygen
20. fibrosis
21. cirrhosis, irreversible
22. microsomal
23. enlarges
24. enlarges, faster
25. narcotic
26. stimulant
27. a. judgement
    b. narcotized.
    e. passes out
    f. stop
28. brain, alcohol, do not
29. water
30. minerals, potassium
31. 1-1/2, alcohol, gulp
32. will not
33. will not

34. liver, breath, urine
35. bloodstream
36. .15
37. 24
38. nervous
39. a.   food, alcohol
     b.   mineral
40. iron, protein
41. hypoglycemia

HIGHLIGHT 8 B: VITAMIN C RUMORS VS. RESEARCH

The purpose of this highlight is:

1. To make you aware of the difficulties in attempting to discover whether a nutrient changes symptoms or _____ a disease.

2. To show you the kinds of research _____ that will have to be _____ before any claim can be proven.

Controls

3. Both groups must be _____ in all respects except for what is being tested.

4. Ideally the control group receives a _____ treatment while the experimental _____ receives a _____ one.

Sample Size

5. The sample size must be large enough to rule out _____ _____.

Placebos

6. The _____-_____ effect must be ruled out.

7. All subjects must believe they are receiving the substance being _____.

8. If an experiment is one in which the subjects do not know whether they are members of the experimental or the control group, it is called a _____ experiment.

Double Blind

9. The _____ must not know which subjects are experimental and which are control subjects so that their reporting, recording, and treatment will not be biased.

10. Repeating an experiment and getting the same results is called _____.

Vitamin C and Cancer

11. Pauling's reports showed that cancer patients receiving vitamin C megadoses live _____.

12. The Mayo study showed that vitamin C _____ (did/did not) help with advanced cancer patients who had received radiation or chemotherapy.

13. If you should decide to take several hundred milligrams a day of vitamin C, you should get it from _____ and vegetables rather than taking _____.

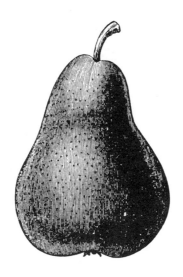

ANSWERS

1. cures
2. questions, answered
3. alike
4. sham, group, real
5. chance variation
6. mind-body
7. tested
8. blind
9. researchers
10. replication
11. longer
12. did not
13. fruits, pills

SELF TEST

1. Which statement best describes the B-vitamins?
    a. They are separate vitamins, with different names, performing distinct functions in the body.
    b. They come together in foods, they work together in the body.
    c. Many of their functions are unknown, and discoveries are made relating to them every few years.

2. B-vitamins are:
    a. absorbed into the lymph system.
    b. absorbed into the bloodstream.
    c. apt to become toxic because of their quick absorption.
    d. a and c
    e. b and c

3. - 7. Matching - B vitamins
    a. destroyed by ultraviolet light rays.
    b. found in many foods in the diet, and deficiencies are unknown.
    c. requires the intrinsic factor for absorption.
    d. can be made in the body from tryptophan.
    e. found in green leafy vegetables; deficiencies are common during pregnancy.

_____ 3. niacin

_____ 4. riboflavin

_____ 5. folacin

_____ 6. vitamin B_{12}

_____ 7. pantothenic acid

8. Insanity is a symptom of an advanced deficiency of this
    vitamin.
    a. vitamin B_{12}
    b. folacin
    c. niacin
    d. vitamin B_6

9. This vitamin is lacking in the diet of strict vegetarians
    (vegans).
    a. vitamin B_{12}
    b. thiamin
    c. riboflavin
    d. niacin
    e. biotin

10. The vitamins involved in the glucose-to-energy pathway are:
    a. niacin, thiamin, pantothenic acid and riboflavin.
    b. niacin, thiamin, vitamin B_6 and B_{12}.
    c. vitamin B_{12}, pantothenic acid and riboflavin.
    d. thiamin, niacin, pantothenic acid and
        vitamin B_6.

11. The breakdown of compounds is called:
    a. anabolism.
    b. catabolism.
    c. metabolism.
    d. two of the above

12. A coenzyme involved in fat synthesis is called:
    a. niacin.
    b. thiamin.
    c. biotin.
    d. pantothenic acid.

13. If a coenzyme forms part of an enzyme structure it is
    called a:

    a. prosthetic group.
    b. an active site.
    c. catabolic participant.
    d. none of the above.

14. The b vitamin involved as part of the coenzymes in amino
    acid metabolism is:
    a. niacin.
    b. pantothenic acid.
    c. vitamin B_6.
    d. vitamin B_{12}.

15. The B vitamin involved in making DNA is:
    a. vitamin B_{12}.
    b. vitamin B_6.
    c. pantothenic acid.
    d. folacin.
    e. none of the above.

16. Aspirin interferes with the following:
    a. the absorption of folacin.
    b. the absorption of vitamin c.
    c. the absorption of iron.
    d. all of the above.
    e. none of the above.

17. The deficiency disease caused by a lack of thiamin is:
    a. pellagra.
    b. beriberi.
    c. scurvy.

18. Especially sensitive to vitamin B deficiency are:
    a. the eyes.
    b. the skin and tongue.
    c. the interstitial tissues.
    d. the hair and nails.

19. Niacin is found in the presence of:
    a. carbohydrate.
    b. fat.
    c. protein.
    d. amylase.

20. Nutrients that are added to enriched breads and cereals
    are:
    a. niacin.
    b. thiamin.
    c. iron.
    d. all of the above

21. Brain cells are designed to use glucose for fuel and need
    niacin and thiamin to convert glucose energy to:
    a. CoA energy.
    b. OH energy.
    c. NAD+ energy.
    d. ATP energy.

22. If your energy requirements are particularly high, _____ is needed in greater amounts.
    a. niacin
    b. riboflavin
    c. thiamin
    d. vitamin B_6.

23. Ultraviolet light can easily destroy:
    a. thiamin.
    b. niacin.
    c. riboflavin.
    d. pantothenic acid.
    e. folacin.

24. Nutrients needed in greater quantity by women taking "the pill" include:
    a. niacin.
    b. vitamin B_6.
    c. folacin.
    d. b and c
    e. a and b

25. Folacin deficiency affects the:
    a. brain and nervous system.
    b. skin and hair.
    c. skin and tongue.
    d. all of the above

26. In order to be absorbed, vitamin B_{12} needs an:
    a. intrinsic factor.
    b. extrinsic factor.
    c. aceytl CoA.
    d. niacin equivalents.
    e. tryptophan.

27. Pantothenic acid and biotin:
    a. are easy to obtain from foods.
    b. are hard to obtain from foods.
    c. should be taken in supplemental form.
    d. have been classified as non-vitamins.

28. Compounds classified as non-B vitamins could include:
    a. pantothenic acid and biotin.
    b. inositol, choline, and lipoic acid.
    c. PABA, bioflavonoids and ubiquinone.
    d. biotin and inositol.
    e. b and c

29. The vitamin C deficiency disease is:
    a. scurvy.
    b. pellagra.
    c. beriberi.

30. In the case of vitamin C, any amount over _____ is considered a megadose:
    a. 500mg.
    b. 1,000mg.
    c. 1g.
    d. 5,000mg.
    e. b and c

31. Vitamin C aids in the absorption of _____ consumed at the same meal.
    a. iron
    b. vitamin A
    c. fatty acids
    d. vitamin D
    e. riboflavin

32. Which of the following foods is not a good source of vitamin C?
    a. broccoli
    b. milk
    c. strawberries
    d. cabbage
    e. cantaloupe

33. The best understood metabolic role of vitamin C is in:
    a. helping to prevent colds.
    b. preventing cancer.
    c. helping to form the protein collagen.
    d. preventing rancidity.

34. Vitamin C is involved in the metabolism of several:
    a. fatty acids.
    b. amino acids.
    c. stress factors.
    d. functions of immunity.

35. Vitamin C interacts with several vitamins and minerals.
    a. true
    b. false

36. Stresses known to increase vitamin C needs are:
    a. infections and burns.
    b. high and low temperatures.
    c. toxic levels of heavy metals.
    d. chronic use of certain medications.
    e. all of the above

37. Proven toxic effects of vitamin C can include:
    a. nausea, abdominal cramps, and diarrhea.
    b. kidney stones.
    c. destruction of vitamin B_{12}.
    d. prevention of cancer.
    e. all of the above

38. An inert, harmless medication given to provide comfort and hope is called a:
    a. prescription.   c. phagocytosis.
    b. blind.   d. placebo.

39. The healing effect that faith in medicine, even inert medicine, often has is called:
    a. control effect.   c. blind effect.
    b. placebo effect.   d. replication effect.

40. An experiment in which the subjects do not know whether they are members of the experimental or the control group is called a:
    a. double blind experiment.
    b. blind experiment.
    c. placebo.
    d. none of the above

41. An experiment in which neither the subjects nor those conducting the experiment know which subjects are members of the experimental group and which are serving as control subjects is called a _____ blind experiment.
    a. single   c. double
    b. triple   d. multiple

42. Repeating an experiment and getting the same results is called:
    a. duplication.   c. triplication.
    b. replication.   d. all of the above

SELF TEST: ANSWERS

ANSWERS

1.   b
2.   b
3.   d
4.   a
5.   e
6.   c
7.   b
8.   c
9.   a
10. a
11. b
12. c
13. a
14. c
15. d
16. d
17. b
18. b
19. c
20. d
21. d
22. c
23. c
24. d
25. a
26. a
27. a
28. e
29. a
30. e
31. a
32. b
33. c
34. b
35. a
36. e

37.   a
38.   d
39.   b
40.   b
41.   c
42.   b

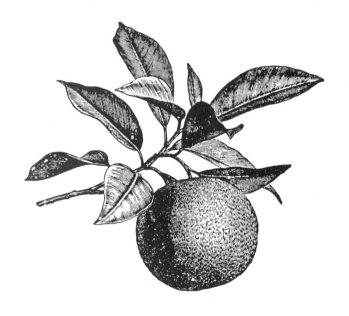

NUTRITIOUS THIRST QUENCHERS

MIXING JUICES

Mixing different citrus juices together can result in some delicious variations. A squeeze of lemon or lime gives sparkle to other juices. You also might try mixing some fresh fruit juice with the frozen or canned juice to improve the flavor and texture. Generally one part just-squeezed juice freshens the flavor of two to three parts prepared juice or fruit drink.

TOMATO "COCKTAIL"

4 cups tomato juice
4 tsp Worcestershire sauce
dash of hot sauce
1/2 cup chopped celery or
   1 celery stick

1 tsp freshly chopped
   parsley (optional)
dash celery salt or table
   salt to taste

Place all ingredients in a blender (1/2 cup celery may be added at this time or a celery stick may be used for a garnish instead); blend for 30 seconds. Divide into 4 equal portions and serve over ice. Makes 4 servings.

PINK TOMATO DRINK

Measure 1 cup tomato juice into container of a blender; add 1/4 cup plain yogurt, a pinch of garlic powder, a pinch of salt and 3 drops Worchestershire sauce. Whirl just until blended. Chill. Serve with green pepper or cucumber garnish.

FRUIT SMOOTHY

Combine 1 cup milk, 1 large banana, 1/4 tsp cinnamon (optional) in a blender and whir until smooth. For extra protein, especially great for breakfast, add a fresh, whole egg. (Be sure you use a fresh, uncracked, clean egg).

Instead of, or in addition to the banana, add strawberries, or a few tbsp of orange or apple concentrate.

FRUIT CHAMPAGNE

6 oz. can frozen, unsweetened apple juice
18 oz. bottle of soda water or sparkling water, etc.

Follow directions on the juice can, using carbonated water instead of tap water. Keep in a bottle or jar with a tight-fitting lid so bubbles won't disappear. Makes about 4 servings of 6 oz. Try other favorite frozen juices.

ORANGE CHILLER

4 cups milk
1-6 oz. can frozen orange juice concentrate

Pour half the milk into a large pitcher or blender. Mix in juice and stir or blend well. Add rest of the milk and add sweetener if you wish. Chill. Shake before using.

CHAPTER 9

The Fat-Soluble Vitamins: A, D, E, and K

YOU WILL LEARN...

1. How vitamin A affects vision.

2. How vitamin A is involved in maintaining mucous membranes throughout your entire body.

3. Other roles of vitamin A including skin, hair and body growth.

4. To understand the danger of overdosing with vitamin A.

5. Which foods provide vitamin A.

6. The important functions of vitamin D in the body.

7. How the body can get vitamin D from sunshine as well as foods.

8. What vitamin E can do for you.

9. What vitamin E cannot do for you.

10. Food sources of vitamin E, and how much you need.

11. Toxicity symptoms of vitamin E and how much is too much.

12. What vitamin K does for you.

HIGHLIGHT 9: WORLD HUNGER

14. The causes of hunger in the developing countries.

15. The scope of hunger in the world and what this means to us.

16. How the problems of hunger can be solved.

17. What we can do now to solve the problem of world hunger.

CHAPTER 9: THE FAT-SOLUBLE VITAMINS

THE FAT-SOLUBLE VITAMINS: A, D, E, AND K

THE ROLES OF VITAMIN A

1. The first fat-soluble vitamin to be recognized was vitamin _____ .

Vision

2. Two kinds of pigment in the cells of the retina are called _____ and _____ . There are also others.

3. A portion of each pigment molecule is the compound _____ .

4. Retinal can only be synthesized if vitamin _____ or its relative are supplied by the _____ .

5. The light-sensitive pigment of the <u>rods</u> in the retina is called _____ .

6. The light-sensitive pigment of the <u>cones</u> in the retina is called, _____ .

7. The _____ are the cells of the retina that respond to light by night.

8. The _____ are the cells of the retina that respond to light by day.

9. In the rods, the protein portion of the visual pigment molecule in rhodopsin is called _____ .

10. Different colors of light are conveyed by a _____ , depending on its wavelength.

CHAPTER 9: THE FAT-SOLUBLE VITAMINS

11. Vitamin A and its relatives in food are the source of all the _____ in the pigments of the eye.

12. Bright light destroys _____.

13. As vital as it is, only _____ of the vitamin A in the body is in the retina.

Maintenance of Linings

14. The membranes composed of cells that line the surfaces of body tissue are called the _____, or mucous membranes.

15. The mucous membranes in the body are so numerous that they line an area within the body larger than a _____ of a football field, and account for most of the body's vitamin _____ need.

16. The normal protein of hair and nails is called _____. Under abnormal conditions cells that normally produce mucus can produce _____.

17. Healthy skin can only be obtained with the help of vitamin _____.

Bone Growth

18. Sacs of degradative enzymes called _____ selectively tear down bone parts not needed so growth can occur.

    Review the list of functions partially dependent on vitamin A in the text.

19. Three different forms of vitamin A are active in the body: retinol, _____, and retinoic acid.

20. Up to a _____ worth of vitamin A may be stored and utilized in the body before deficiencies are noticed.

VITAMIN A DEFICIENCY
Impaired Night Vision

21. Slow recovery of vision after flashes of bright light at night is called _____ _____.

Roughened Surfaces

22. If the cornea of the eye dries due to abnormal mucus production, _____ results.

23. Drying in the mouth leads to decreased appetite and increases _____ .

24. Impaired mucus in the stomach and intestines hinders normal digestion and absorption of _____ as well as causing diarrhea.

25. Increased _____ of the respiratory tract, the urinary tract, and the vagina are probable with a deficiency of vitamin _____ .

26. The hard material accumulating in cells is known as _____ .

Abnormal Growth

27. The primary nutrient deficiency around the world is _____ - _____ malnutrition. The second largest deficiency is vitamin _____ deficiency, causing stunted growth of the skull, abnormal tooth growth, blindness and other abnormalities.

28. Administration of _____ to malnourished children has been seen to result in an epidemic of blindness.

29. Vitamin A depends on _____ and the mineral _____ for its functions and transport.

30. Surveys show that about _____ of people in the United States are getting less than their needs. Widespread deficiencies of vitamin A are caused by a failure to eat _____ .

VITAMIN A TOXICITY

31. Too much vitamin A occurs from taking _____ not from eating _____ .

32. The overdose affects the same systems damaged by a _____ of vitamin A.

33. Alcohol use makes vitamin A toxicity more _____ .

34. Dosages causing toxicity vary but the National Nutrition Consortium advises that adults should avoid intakes of more than _____ to _____ times the RDA to ensure safety.

35. Massive doses of vitamin A taken internally _____ (will/will not) help adolescents with acne.

36. If vitamin A _____ is applied directly to the skin surface acne _____ (may/may not) be helped.

37. Retinol _____ (does/does not) prevent cancer.

    Note to Student: Be sure to understand this important point. Plant foods contain carotene which is converted in the body to true vitamin A. What is not immediately needed is then stored in the liver. If we eat liver, we ingest true vitamin A which the animal or fish has already converted. Supplements contain vitamin A, not carotene. You can only overdose on preformed vitamin A, not from eating vegetables.

    A person drinking excess carrot juice turns yellow because the carotene is being stored in the fat depots but will not suffer toxicity. Toxicity from supplements does not turn you yellow, so there is no visible warning that you are getting too much vitamin A.

38. It is possible to suffer toxicity only when excess amounts of the _____ vitamin from animal foods or supplements are taken.

39. A yellow skin may indicate that _____ is being stored.

VITAMIN A IN FOODS

40. The active form of vitamin A is called _____. Recommended amounts of vitamin A are stated in terms of _____ equivalents. Authorities recommend _____ RE per day for adult men, _____ RE for adult women.

41. The amounts of vitamin A found in _____ are still reported in the old measurement of _____ units (IU) 1 RE is equivalent to _____IU of vitamin A from animal tissues or _____ of vitamin A activity from plant tissues. On the average, 1 RE equals about _____ IU.

42. Any food with significant vitamin A activity must have some
    _____. The green pigment,_____ masks the
    carotene in some vegetables or leafy greens.

43. The process a plant uses to make carbohydrates from carbon
    dioxide and water, using the sun's energy, is called
    _____.

44. Compounds that give color to foods not containing vitamin A
    are called _____. Red cabbage would be an
    example of such a food.

45. The vegetable-fruit group contains many foods that
    contribute vitamin A. Two other groups that offer some
    rich sources are the _____ and _____ group.

46. Another nutrient found in dark-green vegetables is
    _____.

47. Fast foods are notable for their _____ of vitamin A.

ROLES OF VITAMIN D

48. Vitamin A helps to remodel bones, vitamin D helps to
    _____ them.

49. Other nutrients involved in bone building are vitamins
    _____ and _____.

50. Also active in bone building are the hormones,
    _____and calcitonin.

51. The protein collagen and the minerals calcium, phosphorus,
    magnesium, and _____ are also involved in bone
    building.

52. Blood calcium is very active _____.

53. One fourth of the calcium in the blood is exchanged with
    bone _____ every _____.

54. The star of the show is calcium itself, the director is
    vitamin _____.

55. Vitamin D is different from all other nutrients in that the
    body can synthesize it with the help of _____.

56. Therefore, in a sense, vitamin D is not an _____
    nutrient. Rather, it is like a _____.

57. Like other hormones, vitamin D actually enters cells, crosses the membranes of the nucleus and promotes the synthesis of specific _____.

58. The liver manufactures a vitamin D _____ which is released into the blood and circulates to the _____.

59. When ultraviolet rays from the sun hit this compound, it is converted to previtamin _____.

60. Vitamin D even affects _____ secretion in the pancreas.

61. The precursor of vitamin D is made from _____.

62. The chief food source of vitamin D is _____ foods.

VITAMIN D DEFICIENCY AND TOXICITY

63. The vitamin D-deficiency disease in children is called _____.

64. The symptoms of an inadequate intake of vitamin D are those of _____ deficiency.

65. Adult rickets is called _____.

66. An excess of vitamin D causes _____ deposits to form in the soft tissues. This is especially likely to happen in the _____.

67. Pills containing vitamin D should be kept away from _____.

VITAMIN D FROM SUN AND FOODS

68. Animal foods containing a significant amount of vitamin D are _____, liver, and some fish.

69. Milk _____ (does/does not) naturally supply enough vitamin D.

70. Children _____ (can/cannot) depend on sunlight to supply their needs in sunny climates.

71. Overexposure to sun _____ (can/cannot) result in vitamin D toxicity.

CHAPTER 9: THE FAT-SOLUBLE VITAMINS

ROLES OF VITAMIN E

72. One of the main roles for vitamin E is as an
    _____.

73. It is especially effective in preventing the oxidation of
    vitamin _____ and the _____ fatty acids.

74. One of the most important places where vitamin E exercises
    its antioxidant effect is in the _____. At least
    two kinds of cells benefit from the vitamin's protection:
    the red blood cells and the cells of the _____ tissue.

75. Special roles of the vitamin include:
    a. detoxifying _____ _____.
    b. stablizing cell _____.
    c. regulating _____ reactions.
    d. protecting vitamin _____ and polyunsaturated
       _____ _____ from oxidation.

76. Vitamin E may act as a _____ of free radicals.

77. The production of unstable molecules containing more than
    the usual amount of oxygen is called _____.

78. Peroxidation can occur not only in lungs, but also in
    _____ and _____ tissue. Vitamin E seems to exert
    a _____ effect.

79. Vitamin E may have a role in the _____ system and
    protect white cells as well as red cells.

80. Vitamin E _____ (does/does not) affect prostaglandin
    synthesis.

VITAMIN E DEFICIENCY

81. Of 12 possible diseases associated with vitamin E
    deficiency in animals, only _____ has been demonstrated
    in human beings.

82. The vitamin E-deficiency disease in human beings is called
    _____ _____.

83. Abnormal environmental conditions such as _____
    _____ may increase human vitamin E needs.

CHAPTER 9: THE FAT-SOLUBLE VITAMINS

84. Individuals who benefit from vitamin E supplementation are:
    a. _____infants.
    b. People who can't absorb _____.
    c. Individuals with certain _____ disorders.

85. A harmless but painful kind of breast disease which is helped by large doses of vitamin E is called fibro-_____ breast disease.

86. Cramping of the calves of the leg, both when walking and at night is called intermittent _____. This is also _____(helped/not helped) by vitamin E.

87. While science was experimenting with the roles of vitamin E, some things once thought to be helped by vitamin E have been discredited. These include lowering cholesterol, "hot flashes," bladder cancer, preventing heart attacks, improving athletic ability, and restoring or improving _____ _____.

88. Apparently it has no effect on some symptoms of _____ such as wrinkling skin and graying hair.

VITAMIN E TOXICITY

89. Vitamin E _____(does/does not) prevent or cure muscular dystrophy in humans. There is a difference between hereditary muscular dystrophy and _____ muscular dystrophy.

90. Many signs of toxicity are now known or suspected including disturbances of hormonal action, interference with vitamin K, change of blood clotting mechanism, change in blood lipid levels, and impairment of _____blood cell activity.

91. Doses of _____IU are considered megadoses.

VITAMIN E INTAKES AND FOOD SOURCES

92. RDA for vitamin E for adults is _____mg for men, _____mg for women. 1 mg equals 1 IU of D-alpha tocopherol.

93. If a person's polyunsaturated fat intake is high the need for vitamin E is _____(higher/lower).

94. About _____ percent of vitamin E in the diet comes directly or indirectly from _____ _____.

95.   About _____ percent comes from fruits and vegetables, smaller percentages from grains.

96.   The highest concentration of vitamin E is found in wheat germ oil and soybean oil. One of the lowest is _____ oil. Cottonseed, corn, and safflower oil are medium sources.

97.   Vitamin E is easily destroyed by _____ processing and _____.

VITAMIN K

98.   Vitamin K acts on one major body system, the _____ _____ system.

99.   Its presence can make the difference between _____, and _____.

100. One of the main proteins involved in blood clotting is called _____, and vitamin K is essential for its synthesis.

101. Vitamin K is made in the body by _____ _____.

102. Foods containing vitamin K are green _____ vegetables, members of the _____ family, and _____.

103. The bacterial inhabitants of the digestive tract are know as the _____ _____.

104. The RDA is now set at _____ micrograms for vitamin K.

105. People taking _____ drugs may become deficient in vitamin K.

106. The synthetic substitute usually given for vitamin K is called _____.

SUMMING UP

Review summary in text if necessary

ANSWERS

1.   A
2.   rhodopsin, iodopsin
3.   retinal
4.   A, diet
5.   rhodopsin
6.   iodopsin
7.   rods
8.   cones
9.   opsin
10.   photon
11.   retinal
12.   retinal
13.   one-thousandth
14.   mucosa
15.   quarter, A
16.   keratin, keratin
17.   A
18.   lysosomes
19.   retinal
20.   year's
21.   night blindness
22.   blindness
23.   infection
24.   nutrients
25.   infections, A
26.   keratin
27.   protein-kcalorie, A
28.   protein
29.   protein, zinc
30.   one-third, vegetables
31.   supplements, food
32.   deficiency
33.   likely
34.   5, 10
35.   will not
36.   acid, may

37. does not
38. preformed
39. carotene
40. retinol, retinol, 1,000, 800
41. foods, international, 3.33, 10, 5
42. color, chlorophyll
43. photosynthesis
44. xanthophylls
45. milk and meat
46. folacin
47. lack
48. grow
49. C, A
50. parathormone
51. fluoride
52. metabolically
53. calcium, minute
54. D
55. sunlight
56. essential, hormone
57. proteins
58. precursor, skin
59. D3
60. insulin
61. cholesterol
62. animal
63. rickets
64. calcium
65. osteomalacia
66. calcium, kidneys
67. children
68. eggs
69. does not
70. can
71. cannot
72. antioxidant
73. A, essential
74. lungs, lung
75. a. oxidizing radicals
     b. membranes
     c. oxidation
     d. A, fatty acids
76. scavenger
77. peroxidation
78. liver, adrenal, protective
79. immune
80. does
81. one
82. erythrocyte hemolysis

83. air pollution
84.   a.   premature
       b.   fats
       c.   blood
85. cystic
86. claudication, helped
87. sexual potency
88. aging
89. does not, nutritional
90. white
91. 300
92. 10, 8
93. higher
94. 60, vegetable oils
95. 10
96. peanut
97. heat, oxidation
98. blood clotting
99. life, death
100. thrombin
101. intestinal bacteria
102. leafy, cabbage, milk
103. intestinal flora
104. 70-140
105. sulfa
106. menadione

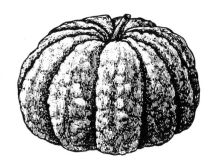

HIGHLIGHT 9:   WORLD HUNGER

1. Hunger wastes the most precious of all the world's resources--the _____ _____.

2. Numerous development programs _____(have/have not) helped malnutrition disappear.

3. The term "hunger" means a continuous lack of the _____ necessary to achieve and maintain health, well being, and protection from _____.

4. It is estimated that there are probably one-half _____malnourished people in the world today.

5. The marks of undernutrition include: Stunted physical _____, swollen _____, _____ irritations, general listlessness and blind eyes.

6. Table I lists _____countries most seriously affected by hunger.

7. The WHO reports that there are _____ million severely malnourished children under the age of five, and another _____ million pre-schoolers suffering from malnutrition.

8. Leila was blind because of a lack of vitamin _____.

9. The most common form of PCM in developing countries is _____growth.

10. The extreme forms of PCM are _____ and _____.

Mother-Child Malnutrition

11. When family food is limited, the first to show the effects
     are: Pregnant or _____ women, and
     _____ children. There are more
     low-_____ babies.

12. Culturally, the last in the family to eat available food is
     the _____.

13. More than 1,300 million people in developing countries do
     not have access to safe _____
     _____.

14. The infant mortality rate is arrived at by calculating the
     number of deaths during the _____year of life per
     _____ live births.

15. A lack of _____ foods causes problems in the
     developing countries. If breastfeeding were to be
     continued along with a simple mixture of grain with peas or
     beans, the infant would thrive.

Food For Growth

16. "Bennimix" consists of rice, sesame and ground
     _____. Benniseed is another name for
     _____.

17. Help is only successful when it meets the _____
     of the people.

18. In Nepal they made a concentrated "super-flour" of
     soybeans, corn and _____ mixed in a 2:1:1
     proportion.

19. A new plant similar to soybeans, cultivated in Southeast
     Asia for years, is the _____ bean plant. It
     can be complemented with _____.

20. It is not enough to know _____,
     malnutrition can only be helped if the new knowledge is
     _____.

Causes of Malnutrition

21. World Hunger _____ (is/is not) the
     result of a world food shortage.

22. The world food problem is economic, technological, environmental and _____ as well as a moral scandal.

23. The question that needs to be answered is not "Why are people hungry" but "Why are people poor?"

Solutions and Alternatives

24. Overpopulation is caused by _____.

25. It _____ (is/is not) possible for us to influence world hunger.

Overpopulation and Hunger

26. The root of the problem is _____. Both hunger and overpopulation are caused by _____.

27. Three factors affect population growth: Birth rates, _____ rates, and standards of _____.

28. Evidence supports the idea that we first have to reduce the _____ _____ rate if we want to reduce the _____ rate.

29. People must feel _____ before they can risk having fewer children.

30. The issues to be addressed in the developing countries are _____, _____, and injustice.

31. In some countries, a large family is a major _____ _____ for the poor.

Distribution of Resources/Land Reform

32. If land is _____ it means it is capable of being plowed and thus food can be grown on it.

HIGHLIGHT 9: WORLD HUNGER

33. The FAO estimates that world food production averages about
     _____ kcalories per person per day, but the
     food is distributed _____.
     a. Huge amounts of grains are fed to
     _____.
     b. _____ of the total food produced is
     lost to pests and spoilage.
     c. Food is distributed _____.

34. The wealthy nations cannot simply give to the
     _____; it weakens them further not to
     _____ for themselves.

35. Four basic needs are required to help the poor nations.
     These are technology, access by the poor to land, knowledge
     and _____. During the development
     period, international _____ _____ is also required.

36. In the 1960's, the Green Revolution, a major agricultural
     effort to help the developing countries
     _____ (failed/succeeded).

37. Which agricultural methods would work best in a developing
     country, labor-intensive or energy-intensive?
     _____

38. Soil _____ is a very serious problem world-wide.
     One process that helps build soil up is _____
     rotation.

Multi-National Corporations: Coordinators of World Hunger?

39. Many observers feel the _____ have
     done more harm than good. A multinational corporation's
     primary concern is _____.

40. It is profitable in poor countries to use land for
     _____ luxuries even while the people suffer
     from hunger.

41. The poor work hard, but they are cultivating crops for
     _____ people rather than for
     _____.

42. One solution to the world food problem is that the
     developed countries should _____ less food away
     from the poor countries rather than giving more food aid.

43. Multinationals also contribute to hunger through inappropriate _____ linking products like Coca-Cola, infant formula and snack foods with health and prosperity.

44. What is needed is an international _____ of conduct.

Lifestyle: Influencing World Hunger

45. Our nation, with _____ percent of the world's population consumes about _____ percent of the world's food and energy resources.

46. Things we could do to change our lifestyle that would have an impact on world hunger would be to:
    a. Consume _____ food.
    b. Depend less on _____-based protein and more on _____-protein.
    c. We could consume _____ energy.

47. Cattle require _____ pounds of grain to produce one pound of meat for our consumption.

Agenda for Action

48. Now is the time to inform our government leaders and corporate policy makers by _____ letters or making our voice heard in other ways.

49. To remain silent is to render _____ to the status quo.

50. After reading some of the suggestions given for personally participating in a project to help end hunger, list three things that you might do right now.

_____

_____

_____

51. Review Table 5 and list several things you might do to reduce energy consumption.

_____

_____

_____

NOTE TO STUDENT: If you have to do a written or oral report for
another class assignment, you might be interested in the
excellent bibliography at the end of this Highlight to give you
ideas for your assignment that will help inform other students
about this issue.

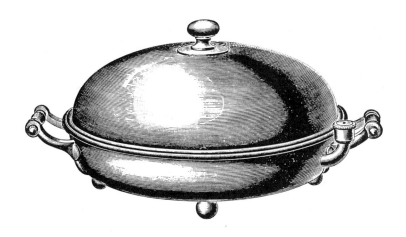

ANSWERS

1.   human being.
2.   have not
3.   nutrients, disease
4.   billion
5.   growth, bellies, skin
6.   44
7.   ten, 240
8.   A
9.   stunted
10. marasmus, kwashiorkor
11. lactating, small, birthweight
12. woman
13. drinking water
14. first, thousand
15. weaning
16. nuts, sesame
17. needs
18. wheat
19. winged, corn
20. why, applied
21. is not
22. demographic
23. given statement
24. hunger
25. is
26. poverty, poverty
27. death, living
28. infant mortality, birth
29. secure
30. poverty, powerlessness
31. economic asset
32. arable
33. 3,000, unequally
     a.   animals
     b.   20%
     c.   unequally

34. poor, fend
35. capital, food aid
36. failed
37. labor-intensive
38. erosion, crop
39. multinationals, profit
40. exportable
41. other, themselves
42. take
43. advertising
44. code
45. six, forty
46.   a. less
       b. animal, plant
       c. less
47. 16
48. writing
49. support
50. student's own ideas
51. student's own ideas

SELF TEST

1. The fat-soluble vitamins include:
    a. A, B, C, and D.
    b. B, C, and E.
    c. A, D, E, and K.
    d. A. B, C. and E.
    e. None of the above

2. Pigments involved in the eye include all <u>but</u> the following:
    a. rhodopsin.
    b. iodopsin.
    c. retinal.
    d. vitamin A.

3. The cells of the retina that respond to light by day are called:
    a. rods.
    b. cones.
    c. circles.
    d. squares.

4. The cells of the retina that respond to light by night are called:
    a. rods.
    b. circles.
    c. cones.
    d. squares.

5. Most of the vitamin A in the body is used to keep the eye functioning properly.
    a. true
    b. false

6. The membranes, composed of cells, that line the surfaces of
    body tissues are called:
    a. urethra.
    b. mucus.
    c. mucosa.
    d. epithelial.

7. Keratin is:
    a. a water-insoluble protein.
    b. the normal protein of hair and nails.
    c. produced under abnormal conditions by cells that
        normally produce mucus.
    d. all of the above
    e. none of the above

8. Three different forms of vitamin A are active in the body:
    a. retinol, retinal, and retinoic acid.
    b. vitamin A_1, A_2, and A_3.
    c. carotene, retinoic acid and pro-A.
    d. retinal, opsin, and **rhodopsin.**

9. The fat-soluble vitamins:
    a. require bile for absorption.
    b. are always part of coenzymes.
    c. are more easily destroyed than are the water-soluble
        vitamins.
    d. a and b
    e. b and c

10. Vitamin A is involved in all but one of the following:
    a. maintaining healthy eye tissues.
    b. maintaining healthy epithelial tissues.
    c. promoting normal tooth spacing.
    d. promoting the laying down of new bone.
    e. protecting chromosomes during cell division.

11. Vitamin A is carried in the blood:
    a. within high-density lipoproteins.
    b. attached to fatty acids.
    c. by a special binding protein.
    d. as a free radical.

12. Vitamin A is stored in the body for as long as:
    a. a week.
    b. a month.
    c. six months.
    d. a year.
    e. it is not stored and must be replenished daily.

13.   Too much vitamin A can be obtained:
    a.   by eating leafy green vegetables frequently.
    b.   by drinking carrot juice daily.
    c.   from vitamin supplements.
    d.   from chicken liver.
    e.   all of the above

14.   Vitamin A activity is measured in:
    a.   retinol units.
    b.   international units.
    c.   retinol equivalents.
    d.   a and b
    e.   b and c

15.   The orange or deep yellow color of vegetables is often caused by:
    a.   xanthophylls.
    b.   chlorophyll.
    c.   carotene.
    d.   all of the above

16.   Massive doses of vitamin A taken internally have been helpful in treating acne.
    a.   true
    b.   false

17.   When a person consuming large amounts of carrot juice turns yellow it is an indication that
    a.   vitamin A toxicity has begun
    b.   the skin is undergoing healthful transition
    c.   carotene is being stored in fat depots
    d.   the liver is overloaded

18.   Skim milk contains just as much protein, calcium, and vitamin A as whole milk.
    a.   true
    b.   false

19.   An adult's RDA for vitamin A is approximately:
    a.   1,000 RE.
    b.   400 IU.
    c.   5,000 IU.
    d.   both a and b
    e.   both a and c

20. Vitamin D could most correctly be called:
    a.   an essential nutrient.
    b.   a hormone.
    c.   a co-enzyme.
    d.   an antioxidant.

21. Vitamin D is involved in everything except:
    a.   insulin secretion from the pancreas.
    b.   the production of proteins.
    c.   calcium homeostasis.
    d.   bones and teeth.
    e.   production of sex hormones.

22. A vitamin D deficiency disease is:
    a.   rickets.
    b.   osteomalacia.
    c.   phosphatase.
    d.   a and b
    e.   b and c

23. Only a few animal foods supply vitamin D. All but one of
    those listed below is rich in vitamin D. The exception is:
    a.   eggs.
    b.   liver.
    c.   fish.
    d.   raw milk.

24. Which of the following foods is not a good source of
    vitamin A or its precursors?
    a.   liver
    b.   spinach
    c.   sweet potatoes
    d.   eggs
    e.   strawberries

25. The active form of vitamin A in vision is:
    a.   opsin.
    b.   collagen.
    c.   dihydroxycholecalciferol.
    d.   retinal.
    e.   keratin.

26. Which of the following is not an important role for vitamin
    A in the body?
    a.   aids in blood clotting
    b.   needed for normal vision
    c.   needed for normal bone growth
    d.   maintains healthy mucous membranes

245

27. Some of our vitamin K requirement is met by synthesis of the vitamin
    a. by intestinal bacteria
    b. from sunlight
    c. from carotene

28. Which of the following surfaces are lined with epithelial cells?
    a. bladder and urethra
    b. mouth, stomach and intestines
    c. eyelids
    d. lungs
    e. all of the above

29. The major sources of vitamin E in the diet are:
    a. meats.
    b. milk and dairy products.
    c. citrus fruits.
    d. vegetable oils.

30. Which of the following is not a role of vitamine E?
    a. detoxifying oxidizing radicals
    b. stabilizing cell membranes
    c. improving endurance in athletic events
    d. regulating oxidation reactions

31. Which of the following is not a role of vitamin E?
    a. curing erythrocyte hemolysis
    b. relieving intermittent claudication
    c. relieving fibrocystic breast disease
    d. preventing heart attacks
    e. protecting red blood cell membranes

32. Anything over _____ IU of vitamin E could be considered a megadose:
    a. 100.
    b. 200.
    c. 300.
    d. 400.
    e. 1,000.

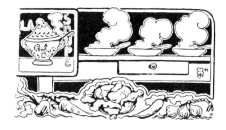

33. Vitamin K is necessary for:
     a.   normal vision.
     b.   normal blood clotting.
     c.   normal bone growth.
     d.   prevention of night blindness.

34. A practice that can seriously interfere with your vitamin K
     status is:
     a.   taking antibiotics.
     b.   eating a poor diet.
     c.   taking sulfa drugs.
     d.   a and c

35. Vitamin K is found normally in:
     a.   green vegetables and milk.
     b.   eggs and cheese.
     c.   whole grains.
     d.   legumes.

TRUE/FALSE (CIRCLE ANSWER)

36. One theory about population growth holds that in many
     countries infant mortality rates are so high that parents
     have a large number of children hoping that some will
     survive to provide them with needed labor and security in
     old age. (true) (false)

37. Shipping food directly to areas where hunger occurs is
     considered to be the ideal way to solve world hunger.
     (true) (false)

38. Many developed nations have long used their land to produce
     food that is exported to industrialized nations, but the
     majority of their own people cannot afford to buy this
     food, even if it were made available for purchase. (true)
     (false)

39. In some circumstances in developing countries, traditional
     farming methods may be more efficient than modern
     agricultural methods. (true) (false)

40. Inequitable distribution of food and of income among the
     population is rarely responsible for malnutrition seen in
     developing countries. (true) (false)

41. Although irrigation can increase the productivity of much
     farmland, intensive irrigation often results in
     accumulation of salt deposits, leading to loss of arable
     land. (true) (false)

CHAPTER 9: SELF TEST

ANSWERS

1. c
2. d
3. b
4. a
5. b
6. c
7. d
8. a
9. a
10. e
11. c
12. d
13. c
14. e
15. c
16. b
17. c
18. b
19. e
20. b
21. e
22. d
23. d
24. e
25. d
26. a
27. a
28. e
29. d
30. c
31. d
32. c
33. b
34. d
35. a
36. T

37.   F
38.   T
39.   T
40.   F
41.   T

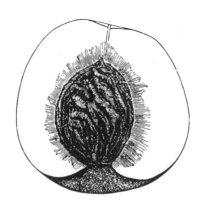

OLD FASHIONED COLE SLAW

1/2 head cabbage, shredded with a knife, salad maker or food processor
1 carrot, grated (optional)
Mix together:

2 tbsp sugar
3/4 tsp salt
few dashes pepper

2 tbsp vinegar
1/4 cup mayonnaise or
    sour cream

  Toss dressing with vegetables, serve cold. Leftovers are good if stored covered.

  <u>Hint:</u> Use half the cabbage for salad and half for our favorite, <u>Panned Cabbage.</u> Coarsely chop cabbage, toss with 1-2 tbsp melted butter in hot skillet. Add 2 Tbsp milk, cover pan and steam for 2-3 minutes until barely tender. A delicious vegetable.

  Use chopped cabbage instead of lettuce in burritos or tacos. It is less expensive than lettuce, and more nutritious.

CARROT LOAF

  Rich in eggs and cheese, this could be a main dish with salad.

About 1 lb carrots
2 large white onions, chopped
1/2 lb very sharp cheddar cheese, shredded
4 eggs, beaten
salt, white pepper to taste

250

Steam carrots and onions or cook in salted, boiling water until carrots are tender. Drain thoroughly and mash. Add cheese and eggs, then salt and pepper to taste. Grease baking dish well then pour in carrot mixture. Place dish in a shallow baking pan with water. Bake at 325° for 1 hour or more. Loaf is ready when it is firm when tested with a knife. Serves 6-8.

STIR-FRIED CAULIFLOWER

1 tbsp vegetable oil
1-1/2 cups thinly sliced celery
2 cups thinly sliced cauliflowerets (about 1 small head)
1 large sweet red or green pepper, thinly sliced
1-2 drops hot pepper sauce

Heat oil in large skillet or wok. Add celery and cook 2-3 minutes, stirring constantly. Add cauliflower and pepper slices. Continue to stir-fry for 4-5 minutes longer. Add seasonings. Mix well, cover, remove from heat and let rest for about 3 minutes before serving.

CHOPPED SPINACH

3 cups cooked spinach   1/4 tsp pepper
1/4 tsp salt   2 tbsp butter
1/8 tsp nutmeg   1/2 cup milk
1 tbsp flour   2 hard-cooked eggs, sliced

Chop spinach very fine and sprinkle with seasonings. Melt butter, stir in flour and cook until smooth. Add spinach and simmer 5 minutes; add milk and cook 3 minutes, stirring constantly. Garnish with egg slices. Serves 6-8.

CHINESE-STYLE VEGETABLES

1 tbsp oil
1 carrot, sliced diagonally
1 stalk celery, sliced diagonally
1/4 green pepper, cut in 1-inch strips
1 tbsp soy sauce, 1 tbsp catsup, 1 tbsp water

Heat oil, add carrots, celery, green pepper and onion slices separated into rings. Cook over medium heat until onion is half cooked, about three minutes. Add soy sauce, catsup and water. Cover and cook over low heat for 10 minutes. (Vegetables should be slightly crisp, overcooking ruins this dish). This is a very tasty combination of vegetables that are available during all seasons.

CHAPTER 10

Water and the Major Minerals

YOU WILL LEARN...

1. That water is the most important "nutrient," making up 50-60% of your body weight.

2. Where water is in the body, the purpose it serves, and how it is regulated.

3. How we take water in, how we excrete it, and the ways the body determines how much is in each body or cellular compartment.

4. The importance of minerals in the water supply.

5. The truth about toxic metals, organic compounds, and other contaminants in our water.

6. How the body's "salts" function in various processes.

7. How minerals contribute to the acid-base balance.

8. What is dangerous about fluid and electrolyte imbalance.

9. Recent findings about high blood pressure and sodium intake.

10. The importance of lifelong adequate calcium intake.

11. The many roles of calcium in the body.

12. Dietary sources of calcium and what to do it you don't drink milk.

13. What chlorine does.

14. The importance of potassium.

15.   About sulfur's association with protein.

16.   How magnesium plays its role.

HIGHLIGHT 10 FOOD ADDITIVES

17.   To understand the terminology and testing procedure relating to intentional food additives.

18.   To put food additives in perspective and not be misled by emotionalism.

WATER AND THE MAJOR MINERALS

1. Every cell in the body is bathed in _____ of the exact composition that is _____ for it.

2. The interstitial fluid always has a high concentration of _____ and _____ ions.

3. The intracellular fluid always has high _____ and _____ concentrations.

4. The entire system of cells and fluids remains in a delicate but firmly maintained state of _____ _____.

5. The amount of salts in our body fluids and their temperature are thought to be the same as the _____ as it was at the time our _____ emerged on land.

6. Water constitutes about _____ to _____ percent of an adult's body weight.

WATER IN THE BODY

7. Water also serves the following functions in the body:
   a. It participates in chemical reactions.
   b. It serves as the _____ for minerals, vitamins, amino acids, glucose.
   c. It acts as a _____ around joints.
   d. It serves as a shock _____ inside the eyes, spinal cord and amniotic sac in pregnancy.
   e. It aids in the body's _____ maintenance.

The constancy of Total Body Water

8. The total amount of water in the body remains _____.

9. _____ governs water intake.

10. One thirst mechanism is in the mouth, the other in a _____ center. The stomach may also play a role.

11. The mechanism of water excretion involves the _____ and the _____.

12. Whenever the body's salt concentration is too high, the hormone _____ is released by the pituitary gland. ADH is an _____ hormone.

13. Water is generated from three main sources:
    a. Water itself.
    b. From _____ we eat.
    c. From the metabolization of the _____ nutrients.

WATER SUPPLY

14. Variables affecting water quality include minerals, heavy metals, _____, and organic compounds. Chlorine and _____ may have been added.

Minerals in Water

15. There are approximately _____ major and trace minerals present in various ground waters.

16. They _____ (can/cannot) make a contribution as nutrients.

17. "Hard" water contains mostly the cations _____ and _____.

18. "Soft" water contains principally _____.

19. Well water can be _____ or _____.

20. _____ water seems to have a more favorable impact on health.

21. The _____ in soft water appears to contribute to a higher incidence of _____ blood pressure and _____ disease.

22. Soft water also may dissolve _____ and _____ from pipes. These minerals can displace _____ from its sites of action in the body.

Toxic Metals in the Water Supply

23. Human technology bears the burden of purifying water contaminated by _____ _____.

24. Metals of greatest concern entering the water supply from toxic wastes from manufacturing processes are _____, cadmium and _____.

25. These metals can change cell membrane structure, alter enzymes, change DNA, cause _____ or birth _____.

26. An element ending up in the water supply is _____ which can accumulate in red blood cells, the _____ and the _____ as well as harm the fetus.

27. Cadmium affects the kidneys, the lungs, and the _____. Cadmium can be absorbed into vegetables and grains eaten by humans.

28. Lowered hemoglobin, intestinal cramps, fatigue and kidney abnormalities might be caused from mild _____ poisoning from automobile exhaust, captured by rain and entering the water supply.

Microorganisms

29. There are three steps involved in treating sewage to make recycled water safe for human use:
     a. primary treatment, b. secondary treatment, and
     c. _____ treatment.

30. Water suitable for drinking is called _____ water. The chemical used in water to kill bacteria is _____.

Organics

31. Organic compounds in water come from sewage, _____, petroleum-based and other industries, and _____ sources.

32. The study of _____ in the water supply is an increasingly important research area.

33.   Bottled water _____ (is/is not) tested for safety and
      required to meet certain standards.

Water quantity

34.   In the future, the water supply may _____ human
      progress.

35.   Processed and fast foods cost _____ (more/less) in
      water and energy than whole foods from the farm.

THE BODY'S SALTS

36.   The most prevalent minerals found in the body are
      _____ and _____.

37.   Four major minerals have major influence on the body's
      water balance. These are: potassium, phosphorus,
      _____ and _____. These form salts that
      are abundant in the body fluids.

38.   Salt is a compound composed of charged particles called
      _____. Positive ions are called _____ and
      negative ions are called anions. Table salt is really
      sodium chloride, symbolized _____.

39.   A solution that can conduct electricity is called an
      _____ solution.

40.   Electrolyte solutions are always _____
      balanced.

41.   A milliequivalent is the number of _____ equal to the
      number of H+ ions in a milligram of _____.

Water Balance

42.   It is useful to remember that "water follows _____."

43.   The force that moves water into a place where a solute is
      concentrated across a divider or membrane, is called
      _____ pressure. Water always flows _____
      the higher osmotic pressure.

44.   Salting lettuce takes _____ out of it, causing it to
      wilt.

CHAPTER 10: WATER AND THE MAJOR MINERALS

Acid-Base Balance

45. In addition to regulating the amount of water in each body compartment, the body uses _____ to regulate the acidity of its fluids.

46. The electrolyte mixtures in the body fluids also protect the body against changes in acidity by acting as _____.

47. A buffer can neutralize both _____ and _____.

Acid-formers and Base-Formers

48. Minerals and foods are either _____-formers or base-formers.

49. Foods are classified as acid or base formers depending on which_____ predominate.

50. Classify which of the following foods are acid or base forming.
    a. Grains _____.
    b. Fruits and vegetables _____.
    c. Meat, eggs, poultry and fish _____.

The Constancy of Total Body Salts

51. Even though a person eats more base-forming foods, or acid-forming foods, the body's total content of electrolytes remains _____.

52. The salt population is regulated by the _____, monitored by the _____ and pituitary glands.

53. The composition of the _____ is affected by what you eat.

54. Another name for kidney stones is _____ _____. They can be either alkaline, made of calcium, or acid such as _____ acid.

55. There are four kinds of taste receptors on the tongue: those sensitive to salt, _____, sour, and bitter flavors.

CHAPTER 10:   WATER AND THE MAJOR MINERALS

Water and Salt Imbalances

56. About 30-45% of the body's sodium is thought to be stored on the surface of the _____ crystals.

57. If you eat a lot of salt, you become _____.

58. Fluid-and-electrolyte imbalances can occur when you _____, or have a prolonged attack of _____.

Note to the student: The person practicing the binge and purge syndrome known as bulimia is often unaware of the seriousness of tampering with the body's electrolyte balance and the effects of dehydration. The bad breath resulting from this has been described as "gross" by friends and associates. The seriousness of the abnormal behavior and results of this practice make one more and more isolated and unattractive when the original purpose may have been to be "slender" and more attractive.

59. Athletes who sweat a lot should know this "rule of thumb": If you have drunk more than about 3 liters (quarts) of water in a day you should take two or more grams of _____ _____ with each additional _____ . Salt tablets are often 1 g each.

60. Another example of fluid loss would be in the case of serious _____.

61. In burns, the loss of fluid is from the _____ space.

Excess Salt

62. People lost at sea will die sooner if they _____ sea water.

63. Another fluid loss situation that can be very dangerous is the taking of self-prescribed _____.

64. The water and salts which we take for granted and usually ignore, are more _____ to _____ than any other nutrients discussed.

SODIUM, OTHER MINERALS, AND HIGH BLOOD PRESSURE

65. Causes of high blood pressure can include _____ of the arteries, _____, and unknown causes.

66. Many studies seem to implicate _____ in relation to high blood pressure.

67. However, people with _____ blood pressure usually do not show an increase when fed large amounts of salt.

68. Some people may be _____ sensitive to sodium and the blood pressure can be lowered by reducing salt intake. People in this group cannot be identified <u>until</u> <u>after</u> they already have high blood pressure.

69. The <u>Goals</u> and the <u>Guidelines</u> both recommend reducing _____ because of this genetic tendency and the fact that many people would benefit without harming others.

70. One mineral that seems to be protective against high blood pressure is _____.

71. In addition, studies show that _____ is low in patients with high blood pressure. The contaminant _____ may contribute to high blood pressure.

72. One gram of salt is about _____teaspoon. If we limited our intake to the recommended 5 grams above and beyond what is naturally in food, that would mean _____ teaspoon.

73. A salty taste is not a reliable guide. A serving of cornflakes contains _____ (more/less sodium) than a serving of cocktail peanuts and chocolate pudding contains _____ more.

<u>CALCIUM</u>

74. Deficiencies of calcium are _____ in human societies.

75. The urgency of obtaining enough calcium has to be learned through _____, because the body sends no signals. Depletion of bone calcium doesn't even show up on an x-ray until it is too late to change it.

76. _____percent of the body's calcium is in the _____.

77. _____percent is in the blood and body fluids.

78. Whenever blood calcium falls too low, three systems are activated to increase it: intestine, bone, and _____.

79. The hormones regulating these systems are
_____ which raises blood calcium and
_____ and thyrocalcitonin which lower it. The
hormone-like vitamin D raises blood calcium by acting at
all three sites listed above.

80. When blood calcium rises above normal it can cause calcium
_____, when it falls too low it can cause calcium
_____.

81. Chronic calcium deficiency depletes the
_____, not the blood.

Roles of Calcium

82. Calcium helps maintain the intercellular cement, or
_____, the transport of _____ in and out of
cells, _____ impulses and assists in blood
_____.

83. Calcium also acts as a _____ with several enzymes,
facilitating chemical reactions.

Calcium Deficiency

84. The calcium deficiency disease in children is called
_____, although lack of vitamin D can also cause it.

85. Adult rickets is called _____, and it means that
the composition of the bones has been altered.

86. Reduced density of the bones is called _____
and a calcium deficiency during the growing years is a
factor always present.

87. An important line of defense against these disorders is a
lifelong _____ intake of _____.

Food Sources of Calcium

88. In Canada and the United States, the recommendation for
adults is _____ to _____ mg per day. High
phosphorus and _____ intakes increase calcium
excretion.

Note to student: The high phosphorus content of soft drinks is thought by some to be responsible for calcium deficiencies in many people.

89. Calcium is found in abundance almost exclusively in a single class of foods--_____ and milk products. If milk as such is not taken, _____ substitutions must be made.

Note to student: it is not acceptable just to do without milk and milk products for any reason without replacing the vital element, calcium, in another way. Study Figure 9 for strategies that work for you.

90. Calcium must be _____ if it is to be absorbed. A high-fat diet may _____(increase/decrease) the absorption of calcium.

91. Hydrochloric acid, vitamin C, some amino acids, and vitamin D _____(aid/inhibit) calcium absorption.

92. Binders preventing calcium absorption are compounds such as _____ acid and _____ acid. Foods such as whole grains, peanuts, rhubarb, spinach and others contain these substances.

93. These binders should not be a problem unless food containing them are _____ in the diet and calcium is in short supply.

94. _____percent of phosphorus is found combined with calcium in the crystals of the bones and teeth. It is called calcium _____.

95. Phosphorus is also part of DNA and _____, the _____ code material present in every cell.

96. Phosphorus also plays many key roles in the cells' transfer of _____. Phospholipids help to transport _____ in the blood and transport _____ in and out of cells.

97. The best source of phosphorus is _____ protein. Extra phosphorus when excreted carries with it some _____.

98. Recommended intakes for phosphorus are the same as for
_____, _____ to 800 mg. per day for
adults. Deficiencies are _____ (common/unknown).

CHLORINE

99. Chlorine is found mostly in association with
_____. It is the major _____ion
of the fluids outside the cells, but it can also move
freely across membranes to balance the _____ of the
blood.

100. In the stomach, the chloride ion is part of
_____ acid, maintaining the strong acidity.

101. The introduction of _____ to public water is one of
the most important public health measures ever introduced.

POTASSIUM

102. _____ is critical to maintaining the
_____.

103. Potassium deficiency affects the _____ cells early,
making a dehydration victim unable to realize water is
needed.

104. All cells must contain _____ and it is also
involved in carbohydrate and _____ metabolism.

105. An early symptom of potassium deficiency is _____
weakness.

106. If a person sweats heavily and often, it is recommended he
or she eat five to _____ servings of potassium-rich
foods each day. The potassium in fruit is used in
_____ building, too.

SULFUR

107. Sulfur is present in all _____ and determines the
shape and contour of the molecules.

108. A high sulfur content is found in skin, hair, and
_____. Deficiency is unlikely if _____ is
adequate.

MAGNESIUM

109.   Most of the body's magnesium is stored in the
_____.

110.   Magnesium also acts in all the cells of the soft
_____ where it is a catalyst for part of the energy
cycle.

111.   Magnesium also helps relax _____ and promotes
resistance to tooth decay.

112.   Deficiency can occur from vomiting, diarrhea,
_____ or protein malnutrition, and in people
using _____.

113.   Magnesium deficit may cause the hallucinations experienced
by _____ during withdrawal from
_____.

114.   The RDA for magnesium is _____ mg for men 300 mg for
women.

SUMMING UP

Review text summary, if necessary. If possible apply this new
knowledge by doing some of the self-study exercises.

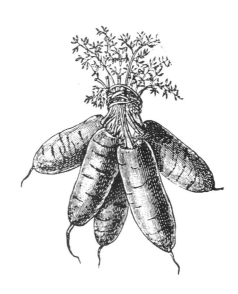

ANSWERS

1.   water, best
2.   sodium, chloride
3.   potassium, phosphate
4.   dynamic equilibrium
5.   ocean, ancestors
6.   55, 60
7.   b.   solvent, minerals
      c.   lubricant
      d.   absorber
      e.   temperature
8.   constant
9.   Thirst
10.   brain
11.   brain, kidneys
12.   ADH, antidiuretic
13.   b.   food
      c.   energy
14.   microorganisms, fluoride
15.   twenty
16.   can
17.   calcium, magnesium
18.   sodium
19.   hard, soft
20.   Hard
21.   sodium, high, heart
22.   cadmium, lead, zinc
23.   human technology
24.   mercury, lead
25.   cancer, defects
26.   mercury, brain, nerves.
27.   bones
28.   lead
29.   tertiary
30.   potable, chlorine
31.   insecticides, other
32.   organics

33.   is
34.   limit
35.   more
36.   calcium, phosphorus
37.   sodium, chloride
38.   ions, cations, NaCl
39.   electrolyte
40.   electrostatically
41.   ions, hydrogen
42.   salt
43.   osmotic, toward
44.   water
45.   ions
46.   buffers
47.   acids, bases
48.   acid
49.   minerals
50.   a. acid, b. base c. acid
51.   constant
52.   kidneys, adrenal
53.   urine
54.   renal calculi, uric
55.   sweet
56.   bone
57.   thirsty
58.   vomit, diarrhea
59.   sodium chloride, liter
60.   burns
61.   intracellular
62.   drink
63.   diuretics
64.   vital, life
65.   hardening, obesity
66.   sodium
67.   normal
68.   genetically
69.   sodium
70.   potassium,
71.   potassium, cadmium
72.   1/5, one
73.   more, even
74.   widespread
75.   education
76.   Ninety-nine, bones
77.   One
78.   kidneys
79.   parathormone, calcitonin
80.   rigor, tetany
81.   bones

82. collagen, ions,
    nerve, clotting
83. cofactor
84. rickets
85. osteomalacia
86. osteoporosis
87. adequate, calcium
88. 700, 800, protein
89. milk, wise
90. soluble, decrease
91. aid
92. phytic, oxalic
93. overused
94. Eighty-five, phosphate
95. RNA, genetic
96. energy, lipids, nutrients
97. animal, calcium
98. calcium, 700, unknown
99. sodium, negative, pH
100. hydrochloric
101. chlorine
102. Potassium, heartbeat
103. brain
104. potassium, protein
105. muscle
106. seven, muscle
107. protein
108. nails, protein
109. bones
110. tissue
111. muscles
112 alcoholism, diuretics
113. alcoholics, alcohol
114. 350

HIGHLIGHT 10: FOOD ADDITIVES

1. All substances are poisons. The right dose differentiates
    a poison and a _____.

2. Many consumers have lost confidence in the safety of the
    _____ _____.

3. There is an important difference between intentional food
    additives and _____ or incidental additives.

Terminology

4. _____ food additives are substances put into
    foods to give them some desirable characteristic.

5. Some additives are _____.

Regulations Governing Additives

6. The agency regulating additives is the _____ and
    _____ Administration, referred to as _____.

7. Before a manufacturer puts a new additive in food, he has
    to prove it is "_____." In addition it must be
    _____ and can be measured in the final food
    product. In addition he has to feed it in large doses to
    _____.

8. The tests are specified and after the petition is filed
    there is a _____ _____ where experts
    present testimony for and against the acceptance of the
    additive.

9. No additives are permanently _____ and the
    regulations specify the amount to be used.

10. Many substances were exempted from _____ with this procedure because there were no known _____ in their use.

11. GRAS stands for "generally recognized as _____" and about _____ additives were on this list. Many of them are being reviewed now that different testing procedures are in use and more facts are known now than previously.

12. Some people feel the _____ Clause is too strict regarding whether or not a substance is a _____.

13. Some feel the amounts necessary to cause cancer are way beyond what human beings would use, but the Delaney Clause states that if the additive causes _____ in animals or humans at any _____ level it cannot be used.

14. If you choose to eat bacon and want to minimize any harm from the nitrites that are added you can do the following:
    a. Consume a food containing vitamin C at the same meal.
    b. Don't fry it too _____.
    c. Don't reuse the bacon _____.

15. Yellow No. 5 (tartrazine) must now be indicated on labels so that consumers may _____ it if they wish.

The Public's Fears about Additives

16. The food packager who advertises "no additives" is not doing the public a _____. He is exploiting the public's _____ rather than helping educate.

17. With improved electronic analytical techniques, additives can now be detected at one part per billion instead of one part per _____, so residues are being found that were overlooked in the past.

Toxicity versus Hazard

18. Toxicity is the ability of a substance to be _____. All substances are _____ if high enough _____ are used.

19. When toxicity is possible under normal conditions of use, it is called a _____.

20. The zone between the concentration normally used and that at which a hazard exists is called the _____ of _____.

Additives in Perspective

21. On the FDA'a list of priority concerns, hazards--in order of concern--are:
    a. Food-born _____, or food poisoning.
    b. Nutrition (many artificial foods do not have it!)
    c. Environmental _____.
    d. Naturally occuring _____ in foods.
    e. Pesticide _____.
    f. Intentional food _____. (Note, this is sixth on the list).

22. If the standards use to test man-made chemicals were applied to "natural" food, fully _____ of the human food supply would have to be banned.

23. Remember, all foods are composed of _____, even if they have no additives in them.

24. The presence of several additives in foods _____ (is/is not) more hazardous than the presence of any one of them.

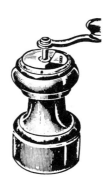

ANSWERS

1. remedy
2. food supply
3. indirect
4. Intentional
5. nutrients
6. Food, Drug, FDA
7. safe, effective, animals
8. public hearing
9. approved
10. testing, hazards
11. safe, 700
12. Delaney, carcinogen
13. cancer, dose
14. crispy, drippings
15. avoid
16. favor, emotionalism
17. million
18. toxic, toxic, concentrations
19. hazard
20. margin, safety
21. a. infection
    c. contaminants
    d. toxicants
    e. residues
    f. additives
22. half
23. chemicals
24. is not

CHAPTER 10:   WATER AND THE MAJOR MINERALS

SELF TEST

1 - 5 Matching - Major minerals
   a.   calcium
   b.   phosphorus
   c.   sodium
   d.   chlorine
   e.   potassium

1. _____ Excessive intakes of this mineral may contribute to the development of high blood pressure in some individuals.

2. _____ This mineral is found in the skeleton, aids in normal blood clotting, and is needed for normal muscle relaxation.

3. _____ Found mainly in the stomach.

4. _____ Aids in maintenance of normal heartbeat. Orange juice and bananas are a good source.

5. _____ Found in the energy-storage compound ATP.

6. The level of calcium in the blood is determined by:
   a.   dietary intakes of calcium.
   b.   calcitonin.
   c.   parathormone.
   d.   all of the above
   e.   (b) and (c) above

7. This disease may be due to inadequate calcium intake during adulthood:
   a.   osteoporosis.
   b.   rickets.
   c.   xerophthalmia
   d.   marasmus.

8. Blood calcium levels can be increased by:
   a.   better absorption of calcium in the intestines.
   b.   retention of calcium by the kidneys.
   c.   release of calcium from the bones.
   d.   all of the above

9. Inadequate levels of calcium in the skeleton may be due to:
   a.   a low protein diet.
   b.   a vitamin D deficiency.
   c.   a vitamin A deficiency.
   d.   a niacin deficiency.

10.   Phosphorus is usually adequate in a diet that contains
      sufficient calcium and protein.
      a.   true
      b.   false

11-14 Matching. How do each of the following affect calcium
absorption in the intestines? (you may use (a), (b) or (c) more
than once.)
      a.   increases calcium absorption
      b.   decreases calcium absorption
      c.   no effect on calcium absorption

11.   _____   The presence of oxalic acid in the same food.
12.   _____   The presence of phytic acid in the same food.
13.   _____   A high need for calcium, such as during pregnancy.
14.   _____   The presence of lactose in the same food.

15.   The percentage of water in the body is about:
      a.   20%.
      b.   40%.
      c.   60%.
      d.   80%.

16.   The part of the brain that regulates thirst is:
      a.   the optic nerve.
      b.   the cerebellum.
      c.   the brain stem.
      d.   the hypothalamus.

17.   The pituitary hormone that regulated kidney retention of
      water is:
      a.   thyroxine.
      b.   ADH (antidiuretic hormone).
      c.   cortisone.
      d.   epinephrine.

18.   About _____ is the minimum amount of water that the body
      must excrete each day to remove wastes.
      a.   200 ml
      b.   400 ml
      c.   900 ml
      d.   2000 ml

19.   Drinking excessive amounts of water can result in excessive
      water retention by the body.
      a.   true
      b.   false

20. Ions that carry a positive charge are called cations.
    a. true
    b. false

21. Which of the following substances is an electrolyte?
    a. water
    b. sodium
    c. a fatty acid
    d. glucose
    e. all of the above

22. The amount and type of electrolytes in the body is largely
    regulated by:
    a. the liver.
    b. the kidneys.
    c. the intestines.
    d. the spleen.

23. Which body contains the most water, considering average
    build?
    a. man
    b. woman
    c. child

24. Which contains the most water,
    a. a slender person?
    b. an obese person?

25. Calcium appears to be involved in:
    a. blood clotting.
    b. cofactor in some enzyme systems.
    c. strengthening bones.
    d. transporting substances in and out of cells.
    e. all of the above.

26. The organ responsible for the greatest water loss to the
    body is the:
    a. kidney.
    b. intestine.
    c. skin.
    d. salivary gland.

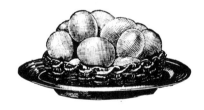

ANSWERS

1. c
2. a
3. d
4. e
5. b
6. e
7. a
8. d
9. b
10. a
11. b
12. b
13. a
14. a
15. c
16. d
17. b
18. b
19 b
20. a
21. b
22. b
23. c
24. a
25. e
26. c

CHILE RELLENOS

2 tbsp butter
5 eggs
1/4 cup flour
1/2 tsp baking powder
dash of salt

4-oz can chopped green chiles
1 cup cottage cheese
1 cup Montery Jack cheese
  grated

Melt butter in a pan. Beat eggs in a large bowl, add flour, baking powder, and salt to eggs. Add melted butter and the rest of the ingredients to the egg mixture. Mix these together and turn back into your pan. Bake at 350° for 35 - 40 minutes. Cut in squares to serve. Can be reheated. Good for breakfast, lunch or dinner.

BROCCOLI WITH CHEESE CASSEROLE

This dish combines two cheeses with eggs and broccoli for a high protein high calcium casserole which can be served as a main dish.

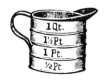

3 eggs
1-8 oz container (1 cup) cottage cheese
1-4 oz pkg shredded cheddar cheese
3 tbsp all purpose flour
1/2 tsp salt
dash of pepper
2 ten-oz pkgs frozen chopped broccoli, thawed or an equivalent amount of fresh which has been lightly steamed and chopped.

Preheat oven to 350 degrees. In a large bowl beat eggs slightly with a wire whip or fork; beat in both cheeses, flour, salt and pepper. Drain broccoli well. Stir into egg mixture. Pour into a greased 9" x 9" pan, spreading evenly into pan with a spoon. Bake 350°-35 minutes till mixture is firm and pulls away from sides of the pan. Serve immediately. 6-8 servings.

RECIPES YOU CAN TRY...

EASY CUSTARD FROM DRY MILK
(Cooked on top of the stove)

2 eggs   2 cups hot water
1/4 cup sugar   1 tsp vanilla
2/3 cup dry milk powder
1/4 tsp salt

   Break the eggs into a bowl, beat slightly and add the
sugar, dry milk, salt, and flavoring. Add hot water a little
at a time and blend well.

   Pour the mixture into custard cups or baby-food jars.
Cover the cups with foil or the jars with lids. Sprinkle with
nutmeg or cinnamon (or both) as desired. Place a towel or large
potholder or rack on the bottom of the pan. Set the cups of
custard on the rack or towel and fill the pan with <u>cold</u> water to
a depth of one-half the height of the cups or jars.

   Put a tight cover on the pan and bring the water to a boil.
Turn off heat. Steam for 10 minutes. The custard is done when
a knife blade put down into the middle comes out clean and not
milky looking. If not done, heat the water and leave a few
minutes longer. Take the cups out of the pan and let them cool.

   This custard may also be baked in the oven. Pour custard
into a pan and set it into a larger pan of hot water. Bake in
moderate oven, 325°, for about 1 hour. Yield: 6 servings,
90 calories per serving.

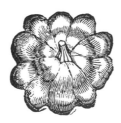

CHAPTER 11
The Trace Minerals

YOU WILL LEARN...

1. About the intricate interrelationships of trace minerals in the body.

2. The importance of iron, what processes in the body it is involved in, and what happens when you are deficient.

3. Where there are sources of iron in the diet, and what happens if you get too much.

4. About important new research in zinc--where you get it, how you lose it, and whether it can be toxic.

5. The interesting history of iodine brought up to date.

6. About the vital roles of copper.

7. That manganese can be dangerous.

8. How fluoride can help more than teeth.

9. That chromium can be involved in diabetes and carbohydrate metabolism.

10. How selenium has been linked with cancer prevention.

11. About molybdenum's link with protein.

12. That silicon, tin, vanadium, cobalt, silver, mercury, lead, barium, arsenic and others may play key roles in human health.

HIGHLIGHT 11: CONTAMINANTS IN FOOD AND WATER

13. About the concern for indirect additives, both heavy metals and organic halogens.

14. What research has proven about lead, mercury, and DDT.

15. To see contaminants in perspective.

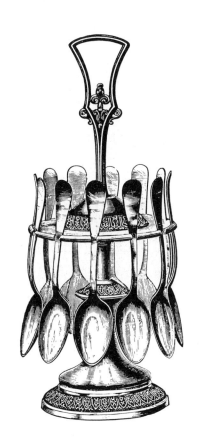

THE TRACE MINERALS

1. All the trace minerals in the body would hardly fill a
    _____.

2. The way you _____ and the way the body handles these
    _____ enables you to maintain health.

3. The best known trace elements are_____, _____ and
    _____.

4. Until recently, _____ deficiencies were unheard of.

IRON

5. Iron is a problem nutrient for _____ of people. To
    prevent deficiencies you must be _____ _____.

Iron in the Body

6. Iron is found in every _____ in all _____
    _____.

7. Most of the iron in the body is part of the proteins
    _____ and _____.

8. Hemoglobin is the oxygen-carrying protein of the
    _____ cells; myoglobin the oxygen-carrying
    protein of the _____ cells.

9. The average red blood cell lives about _____
    months. The iron is _____ through each new
    generation.

10. Iron is lost in urine, _____, and shed
    _____. Iron loss is greatest whenever
    _____ is lost.

280

CHAPTER 11:   THE TRACE MINERALS

11.   Iron is carried to tissues throughout the body by
      _____, a blood protein.

12.   The storage proteins for iron are _____ and
      hemosiderin.

13.   Normally only about _____ percent of dietary iron is
      absorbed.

14.   Women are at risk for iron deficiency because of monthly
      menstruation and possible _____.

Iron-Deficiency Anemia

15.   Smaller cells in the blood that are lighter red than usual
      and pale skin or fingernails are beginning symptoms of
      _____-deficiency anemia. Because oxygen is reduced,
      _____ is limited and symptoms of
      _____,weakness, headaches, and apathy appear.

16.   Other body tissues are also affected, especially the
      _____. Reduced IQ, _____ and other
      psychological disturbances may appear.

17.   A craving for unnatural substances such as ice, clay,
      starch and other nonnutritious substances is called
      geophagia or _____.

18.   Another tissue sensitive to depletion of iron stores is
      _____ tissue, greatly affecting work capacity.

19.   When seeking a solution to behavioral problems, check the
      adequacy of the _____.

20.   The body's iron status is determined by measuring the
      amount of _____. The normal level is 14 to 15
      g/1000 ml for adult men, 13 to 14 g/1000 ml for women.

21.   Because nutrients depend on one another, a low hemoglobin
      may be caused by iron deficiency but also from too little
      vitamin _____, vitamin E, vitamin B , or vitamins
      A and C.

22.   The Boston study of people with low hemoglobin levels
      showed that _____ made a difference, supplements
      did not.

CHAPTER 11:   THE TRACE MINERALS

Iron Overload

23. Unneeded iron is captured by a _____ block in the intestinal cells.

24. Two kinds of iron overload are known. One is caused by ingesting too much iron, the other is a _____ defect. Drinking _____ increases the absorption of iron.

25. Iron overload is more common in _____ than _____.

26. As few as _____ tablets of iron supplements have caused death in a child.

Iron in Foods

27. The usual Western mixed diet provides only about _____mg. of iron in every 1,000 kcalorie. The iron RDA for women is _____ to _____ mg. per day. It is difficult to meet a woman's iron needs because of restricted calories.

28. The iron in different foods is absorbed differently by the body. The Monsen system indicated an absorption rate of _____ percent in meat-fish-poultry and soybeans. Less than _____ percent from eggs, whole grains, nuts and dried beans. Only two percent of iron from _____ is absorbed.

29. Vitamin _____ eaten with any iron source doubles or _____ the amount of the iron absorbed.

30. The iron-holding part of the hemoglobin and myoglobin proteins is called _____. _____ iron is much more absorbable than _____ iron.

31. Foods in the milk group are _____ (good/poor) sources of iron.

32. Use of an iron skillet _____ (enhances/destroys) iron status.

33. The iron in iron-fortified foods is _____ (well/poorly) absorbed.

34. At present _____ percent of all iron consumed in the United States is from fortified foods. Fortification means adding _____ to food, but not necessarily the nutrients originally found in it. (Example: adding iodine to salt.)

ZINC

35. Zinc has only been identified as being important during the last _____ years.

Zinc in the Body

36. Zinc appears in every body _____ but is not present in the same amounts.

37. Zinc is found in abundance in the eye, liver, kidney, muscle, _____, skin, and male reproductive organs.

38. There are more than _____ known enzymes which require zinc as a _____.

39. Zinc is necessary for normal metabolism of the energy nutrients and _____. It is associated with the hormone _____ in the pancreas. It is involved in the synthesis of DNA and _____, cell replication, immune reactions, taste, perception, and more.

40. Extra zinc is held within the _____ cells, and only the amount needed is released.

41. While traveling in the bloodstream, zinc is transported by _____.

42. An interesting phenomenon in zinc nutriture is the _____ of zinc in the body.

43. People who take supplements of _____ acids may interfere with their zinc_____.

44. Losses of zinc occur from alcohol abuse, during fasting or injury, from lost sweat, menstrual blood, seminal fluid and human _____.

Zinc Deficiency and Toxicity

45. In the 1960's it was observed that zinc deficiency caused growth retardation and arrested _____ development.

46. More recently, children in the U.S. who were "picky eaters"
     showed poor growth, poor appetite, and decreased
     _____ sensitivity.

47. Zinc deficiency can cause a vitamin _____ deficiency
     because of its interaction. Lack of zinc also delays
     _____ healing.

48. Vegetarians, dieters, pregnant females--especially
     teenagers--the elderly and infants and children still
     growing may be at risk for _____ deficiency. A diet
     of 1500 calories per day only provides _____ percent of
     the RDA for zinc.

Zinc in Food

49. Foods of high _____ content provide zinc, especially
     oysters and liver.

50. People who consume the Basic Four probably _____
     (will/will not) get enough zinc.

51. Substances interfering with the availablility of zinc for
     absorption include _____ acid, calcium, phosphorus and
     _____. Zinc is mostly removed in the
     refining of grains.

52. Whole grains have _____ (more/less) <u>available</u> zinc
     than refined grains.

53. The fermentation of yeast is _____
     (favorable/nonfavorable) in destroying phytate which binds
     zinc.

IODINE

54. Iodine is part of the _____ hormone.
     _____ controls the rate at which energy is
     released.

55. An enlarged thyroid gland is called a _____.
     Ninety-six percent of these cases are caused by
     _____ deficiency, and 4% by the overconsumption of
     plants of the _____ family.

56. An iodine-deficiency disease of mental and physical
     retardation is called _____.

CHAPTER 11:   THE TRACE MINERALS

57. It is important for most people who live in the Plains states to use _____ salt.

58. Most people get enough iodine by consuming _____ or vegetables grown in soil that contains iodine.

59. There is a/an _____ (decrease/increase) in available iodine in the U.S. food supply.

Note to student: Iodides are commonly used in restaurants and fast food chains as a sanitizing agent and some researchers feel that this is contributing to the overall increase in iodine.

COPPER

60. The body contains about _____mg. of copper, which performs several vital roles.

61. Copper is part of several _____ and is a _____ in the formation of hemoglobin.

62. Copper is also involved in the manufacture of _____ and the _____ of wounds. It helps maintain the _____around nerve fibers and is involved with the mineral _____ in electrical impulses related to respiration and the release of _____.

63. Copper deficiencies are _____ (rare/common).

64. Food sources of copper include grains, shellfish, organ meats, legumes, fruits and _____. About _____ of the copper taken in food is absorbed.

MANGANESE

65. Even 20 mg. of manganese represents _____ of molecules.

66. Manganese deficiency in animals affects the _____, reproduction, the nervous system, and _____ metabolism.

67. One must be careful not to take too many _____ containing trace minerals.

68. A real danger with manganese is_____.

CHAPTER 11: THE TRACE MINERALS

FLUORIDE

69. Fluoride has to do with strengthening the _____ and teeth.

70. Drinking water is the usual source of _____ but _____ and _____ may supply substantial amounts.

71. About _____ million people are drinking fluoridated water.

72. Fluoride may be helpful for older adults by helping to prevent _____.

73. A mottling of the tooth enamel due to taking in too much flouride during tooth development is called _____.

CHROMIUM

74. Chromium works closely with the hormone _____. When chromium is lacking a _____-like condition results.

75. GTF means _____ _____ _____.

76. GTF is a small organic compound containing _____.

77. Depleted chromium stores are linked to adult-onset _____ and _____ failure in children that are malnourished. Chromium has also improved faulty _____ metabolism is groups of older people.

78. GTF has been purified from _____ yeast and pork _____ and is probably present in other foods.

SELENIUM

79. Selenium is found as part of larger molecules, especially certain _____. It is also an _____ and can substitute for vitamin _____ in certain functions.

80. Selenium deficiency affects the _____. Heart disease caused by selenium deficiency is named _____ disease.

CHAPTER 11: THE TRACE MINERALS

81. Dietary _____ adequacy may be one of the many
     health factors that defend against _____.
     However, it hasn't been proven that selenium _____
     will prevent cancer.

MOLYBDENUM

82. Molybdenum is part of the giant _____ molecules.

83. Deficiencies of molybdenum are _____ (known/unknown).

84. Too much molybdenum causes _____ in animals.

OTHER TRACE MINERALS

85. None of the trace minerals has been know for _____
     _____.

86. Nickel is important for the health of many body
     _____.

87. Silicon is involved in bone _____.

88. Tin is necessary for _____ in animals and probably
     humans.

89. Vanadium is necessary for growth, bone _____ and
     normal _____.

90. Cobalt is the mineral in the large vitamin _____
     molecule, which is named _____.

91. The roles of silver, mercury, lead, barium, arsenic and
     _____ are being studied.

92. The most important facts being discovered about trace
     minerals are the _____ between them.

ANSWERS

1. teaspoon
2. eat, minerals
3. iron, iodine, zinc
4. zinc
5. millions, well informed
6. cell, living things
7. hemoglobin, myoglobin
8. blood, muscle
9. four, recycled
10. sweat, skin, blood
11. transferrin
12. ferritin
13. ten
14. pregnancy
15. iron, energy, fatigue
16. brain, hyperactivity
17. pica
18. muscle
19. diet
20. hemoglobin
21. B_6 22. food
23. mucosal
24. hereditary, alcohol
25. men, women
26. 6-12
27. 5-6, 14, 18
28. 40, 10, spinach
29. C, triples
30. heme, Heme, nonheme
31. poor
32. enhances
33. poorly
34. 25, nutrients
35. ten

36. tissue
37. bones
38. 70, cofactor
39. alcohol, insulin, RNA
40. intestinal
41. proteins
42. recycling
43. amino, absorption
44. milk
45. sexual
46. taste
47. A, wound
48. zinc, 40
49. protein
50. will
51. phytic, fiber
52. more
53. favorable
54. thyroid, thyroxin
55. goiter, iodine, cabbage
56. cretinism
57. iodized
58. seafood
59. increase
60. 75-100
61. enzymes, catalyst
62. collagen, healing, sheath, iron, energy
63. rare
64. vegetables, 1/3
65. billions
66. bones, fat
67. supplements
68. toxicity
69. bones
70. fluoride, fish, tea
71. 100
72. osteoporosis
73. fluorosis
74. insulin, diabetes
75. glucose tolerance factor
76. chromium
77. diabetes, growth, carbohydrate
78. brewer's, kidneys
79. enzymes, antioxidant, E
80. heart, Keshan
81. selenium, cancer, supplements
82. protein
83. unknown
84. toxicity

85. very long
86. tissues
87. calcification
88. growth
89. development, reproduction
90. B_{12}, cobalamin
91. cadmium
92. interactions

CONTAMINANTS IN FOOD AND WATER

1. Indirect additives are a matter for _____ concern.

2. In 1953, 121 people in Japan suffered from _____
    poisoning.

3. Another heavy metal causing problems in the United States
    and other places is _____.

4. An example of an organic halogen is _____.   An
    insecticide that became widely used and was linked to many
    problems is _____.

Lead

5. Lead affects the tissues of the nervous system,
    _____ and bone _____ as well as the fetus.
    Children are even more vulnerable than adults.

6. Again, you can see how interconnected _____ is
    with the effect of contaminants.

7. Healthy, well-nourished animals are used for
    _____.   This might affect the results of the
    "maximum _____ level" of a contaminant.

8. Unsupervised chelation "therapy" may remove the wrong
    _____.

DDT

9. DDT finds its way into stored _____ or oil depots of
    animals or _____.

10. In studying contamination, it is the _____ that makes
    the difference.

HIGHLIGHT 11:   CONTAMINANTS IN FOOD AND WATER

11.   Human milk has _____ (more/less) DDT than cow's milk.

12.   Some additives, such as _____ may actually be beneficial.

13.   DDT's toxicity depends on the state of _____ of the animal.

Perspective on contaminants in foods

14.   There seem to be a lot of unanswered _____ in the search for answers about long-term effects of some substances.

15.   People working on the problem need to have an in-depth understanding of _____.

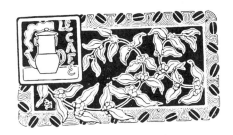

ANSWERS

1. real
2. mercury
3. lead
4. PBB, DDT
5. kidney, marrow
6. nutrition
7. experiments, permissible
8. ions
9. fat, plants
10. amount
11. more
12. BHT
13. health
14. questions
15. nutrition

CHAPTER 11: THE TRACE MINERALS

SELF TEST

1. Body sodium levels are largely regulated through:
   a. changes in intestinal absorption, depending on need.
   b. changes in fecal excretion.
   c. storage of excess sodium in the liver.
   d. excretion of excess sodium by the kidneys.
   e. all of the above

2. Fruits are quite high in sodium
   a. true
   b. false

3 - 6 Matching
   a. iodine   b. chromium   c. zinc
   d. fluoride   e. copper

_____ 3. Deficiency symptoms include a loss of taste, and underdevelopment of the sexual organs.
_____ 4. A deficiency results in goiter.
_____ 5. Adequate levels of intake greatly reduce the amount of tooth decay.
_____ 6. Found in a larger molecule called Glucose Tolerance Factor.

7. A very poor source of iron is:
   a. legumes.
   b. dried fruits.
   c. whole grain breads.
   d. milk.

8. When the natural fluoride content of a water supply is a little too high, it may cause:
   a. death.
   b. paralysis.
   c. cancer.
   d. mottling or discoloration of tooth enamel.
   e. goiter.

CHAPTER 11:   THE TRACE MINERALS

9. A person consuming a balanced diet supplying 2000 kcalories
   a day can expect to get about:
   a. 4 milligrams of iron a day.
   b. 6 milligrams.
   c. 12 milligrams.
   d. 30 milligrams.

10. Which of the following foods is the best source of available
    iron?
    a. Spinach.
    b. Hamburger.
    c. Rice.
    d. Peas.

11. An example of a toxic metal that pollutes some water is:
    a. zinc.
    b. calcium.
    c. mercury.
    d. sodium.

12. Iron is a component of:
    a. hemoglobin.
    b. myoglobin.
    c. many vital proteins.
    d. a and b
    e. all of the above

13. The percentage of iron in the blood is about:
    a. 50 percent.
    b. 80 percent.
    c. 25 percent.
    d. 100 percent.

14. Which of the following is a storage form of iron?
    a. Ferritin.
    b. Transferrin.
    c. Heme.
    d. Trabeculae.

15 - 18 Matching - Iron-containing compounds.
    a. ferritin   b. myoglobin
    c. transferrin   d. hemoglobin

_____ 15. Carries oxygen in the bloodstream.
_____ 16. Holds oxygen in the muscle cells.
_____ 17. One of the major forms iron is stored in.
_____ 18. Transports iron from the intestine to the liver and
           bone marrow.

19. Normally, _____ of the dietary iron is absorbed from the
     intestine.
     a. about 10 percent
     b. about 20 percent
     c. about 30 percent
     d. about 40 percent
     e. about 50 percent

20. The major symptom of an iron deficiency is:
     a. night blindness.
     b. abnormal blood clotting.
     c. anemia.
     d. a skin rash.

21. Iron deficiency may cause some people to crave things such
     as clay and ice. This ingestion of non-nutritious
     substances is known as:
     a. tetany.
     b. pica.
     c. hemosiderosis.
     d. goiter.

22. Heme iron is found in which of the following?
     a. Fruits high in vitamin C.
     b. Deep yellow vegetables.
     c. Green, leafy vegetables.
     d. Meats, poultry, fish.

23. Cretinism is a severe manifestation of manganese
     deficiency.
     a. true.
     b. false.

24. Among the richest sources of chromium are white flour,
     white sugar, butter and margarine.
     a. true
     b. false

25. Sea salt is a better choice than store salt in a region
     where goiter is a risk.
     a. true
     b. false

26. The best food sources of copper include grains, shellfish,
     organ meats, legumes, dried fruits, fresh fruits, and
     vegetables.
     a. true
     b. false

27. Selenium-poor soil may correlate with certain kinds of cancer.
    a. true
    b. false

28. An individual with low iron stores, compared with one with high iron stores, absorbs _____ percentage of iron from foods.
    a. a higher
    b. a lower
    c. an equivalent

29. Which of the following does not aid in absorption of nonheme iron?
    a. Drinking tea with a meal
    b. An undefined "meat factor" in meat
    c. An acid medium near the absorption site
    d. Cooking acid foods such as tomatoes in an iron utensil before consuming them

30. _____ aids in the absorption of nonheme iron.
    a. Riboflavin
    b. Vitamin B6   c. Vitamin C
    d. Vitamin K

31. The form of nonheme iron that is most easily absorbed is _____ iron.
    a. Ferrous
    b. Ferrite
    c. Ferritous
    d. Ferric

32. People who routinely consume diets containing large amounts of _____ may have low chromium intakes.
    a. bran and germ from whole grains
    b. beef and pork
    c. cheese and brewer's yeast
    d. refined grain products and sugars

33.   _____ is currently under study as one possible means
of treating osteoporosis.
   a.   Zinc
   b.   Fluoride
   c.   Iodine
   d.   Selenium
   e.   Copper

34.   _____ is an intergral part of enzymes in the body that
are involved in hemoglobin production, in the electron
transport system, and in normal development of connective
tissue proteins in arteries and bones.
   a.   Zinc
   b.   Iron
   c.   Copper
   d.   Selenium
   e.   Chromium

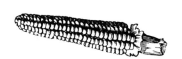

ANSWERS

1. d
2. b
3. c
4. a
5. d
6. b
7. d
8. d
9. c
10. b
11. c
12. e
13. b
14. a
15. d
16. b
17. a
18. c
19. a
20. c
21. b
22. d
23. b
24. b
25. b
26. a
27. a
28. a
29. a
30. c
31. a
32. d
33. b
34. c

BAKING WITH WHOLE WHEAT FLOUR...

White flour should be called "impoverished" instead of "enriched." Many trace minerals are removed and never replaced. The nutrition-conscious cook can learn to make everyday meals more wholesome by serving whole grains.

Get Off To The Right Start

Store-bought whole wheat flour has already been degerminated and may be stale. The flavor and nutrition do not compare in any way to freshly-ground wheat flour. You may be able to find a store or group which will sell you freshly ground whole wheat flour. The Nutrition Club at Cuesta College grinds and sells whole wheat flour to students and townspeople at reasonable cost as a special project.

STORING

Treat your whole-wheat flour as a fresh food to preserve both nutrients and flavor. Store in a closed container in the freezer for long storage, or in the refrigerator if it will be used in a few weeks. (Flour does not have to thaw before using).

SPECIAL HELPS

Start out by substituting whole wheat flour for half or even less of the unbleached or white flour called for in your favorite recipes. The proportion can be increased as tastes in your family change. Depending on moisture content of recipe, often one to two tbsp less flour per cup is needed.

Following are some recipes that will be successfull if you start with good flour.

RECIPES YOU CAN TRY...

BUTTERMILK PANCAKES

Mix 1 cup whole wheat flour with 1 tsp soda and a dash of salt. Stir in 1 egg, 1 cup buttermilk and 3 tbsp oil. Mix and bake on ungreased hot griddle until browned, turning once.

BANANA BREAD

2 large or 3 small bananas
1/2 cup shortening
1 cup sugar
1/2 tsp. salt
2 cups whole wheat flour
1 tsp. baking soda

2 eggs
3 tbsp buttermilk
(or just add 1/2 tsp. vinegar
to regular milk to total the
3 tbsp)
1/2 cup nuts, optional

You can use very ripe or soft bananas, but cut out any black spots first. Cream the bananas in a bowl, add the shortening, sugar, eggs and salt. Beat until fluffy and blended. Add the flour, soda and buttermilk (or soured milk) and beat just until smooth. Stir in nuts and turn batter into a greased 9 x 5 inch loaf pan and bake at 350° for about 1 hour. Test middle with clean toothpick to be sure it is done. Recipe can be doubled and extra loaf frozen.

ZUCCHINI BREAD

3 eggs
3/4 cup oil
1 tsp cinnamon
1 tsp soda
2 cups grated zucchini
1 cup white flour

1-2/3 cups brown sugar
1 tsp vanilla
1 tsp salt
1/4 tsp baking powder
2 cups whole wheat flour
1 cup chopped nuts, optional

Beat eggs until foamy in mixing bowl. Add sugar, oil, vanilla, cinnamon, salt, soda, baking powder, zucchini and flour; mix well. Turn batter into greased 9 x 5 inch loaf pan and bake at 350° for 1 hour and 20 minutes. Remove from pan and cool on rack.

CHAPTER 12

Nutrition Status, Food Choices, and Diet Planning

YOU WILL LEARN...

1. What is involved in nutrition assessment.

2. What nutrition assessment can and cannot tell you.

3. Important information about computer and hair analysis.

4. How well we dc eat.

5. What surveys were done and what they tested for.

6. The importance of identifying nutrient deficiences.

7. Why we eat the food we do.

8. How to plan the ideal diet for yourself.

9. The best way to use new foods.

10. What it takes to be a healthy person.

    HIGHLIGHT 12: THE NEW FOODS AND NUTRITION LABELING

13. What you need to know to make the best choices of food at the market.

14. What all the labeling laws are about and how to use the information to your advantage.

15. What labels say, and don't say, and how information can be misleading to the uninformed.

NUTRITION STATUS, FOOD CHOICES, AND DIET PLANNING

1. Food does not become nutrition until it passes the
    _____.

NUTRITION ASSESSMENT

2. Nutrition assessment involves making an inventory of
    nutrition _____ and liabilities as determined by
    four techniques:
    a. history _____
    b. anthropometric _____
    c. physical _____
    d. biochemical _____

Historical Data

3. A person's _____ reveals many clues about his present
    nutrition status.

4. Circumstances of a person's life such as environment, his
    _____ facilities, previous _____, who he
    associates with, and others have an impact on nutrition
    status.

Note to student: Consult Table 12-1 and Appendix E for
information on recording assessment of nutrition status.

5. A commonly used method of obtaining food intake data is the
    24-hour _____.

6. Another method is to obtain a "_____ intake
    pattern."

7. Another approach is the food frequency _____.

8. A food _____ works well with cooperative patients. Other important information needed for behavior modification can also be obtained at this time.

9. Food intake data can then be compared to standards such as the _____.

10. Sufficient intake of a nutrient does not _____ adequate nutrition status for an individual.

Anthropometric Measures

11. Anthropometrics are _____ measurements that reflect growth and _____.

12. Measurements are compared with _____ derived from large numbers of people with similar backgrounds.

13. Examples of anthropometrics would be height and _____.

Physical Examination

14. Physical signs of malnutrition appear most rapidly in places such as the hair, _____ and gastrointestinal _____.

Biochemical Tests

15. Common biochemical tests include blood and _____, but others are used to assess protein nutrition.

16. An indicator of lean body mass is the test for_____ excretion.

17. An abnormal lab value for one nutrient may reflect abnormalities of other _____ in the body.

Assessment of PCM

18. If a person's visceral _____ is depleted but his body protein and fat are adequate, he has _____.

19. Counting lymphocytes (white blood cells) and testing skin antigens are two ways of testing the _____ system. These may be helpful in diagnosing PCM.

CHAPTER 12:NUTRITION STATUS, FOOD CHOICES, AND DIET PLANNING

Nutrition Assessment Completed

20. Computers _____ (can/cannot) accurately assess your nutrition status.

21. Food composition data _____ (is/is not) complete for all vitamins, minerals, and fiber.

22. Protein status _____ (can/cannot) be determined by hair root analysis.

23. No trace minerals except zinc _____ (can/cannot) reliably be assessed by hair analysis.

24. If a person is called a "nutritionist," you _____ (can/cannot) be sure he or she is competent to administer tests to determine your nutrition status.

HOW WELL DO WE EAT?

25. In the 1930's, it was determined that at least _____ of the population might be poorly fed.

26. Programs to correct our nutrition include:
    a. The _____ Act of 1936.
    b. The National _____ _____ Program.
    c. Adding _____ to salt.

27. Nutrients found lacking in many surveys were the minerals _____ and _____, the B vitamins _____ and _____ vitamin A, and _____. Note: other nutrients now known to be important were not studied at all in early surveys.

The Ten State (National Nutrition) Survey

28. This survey included _____ people.

29. It involved not only food intake but also _____ tests, physical _____, anthropometric _____, and _____ histories. Other factors such as ethnic background and available foods were also considered.

30. Low-income and uneducated people had _____ nutrition in every respect. Wealthy people could also have _____ nutrition.

31. The mineral _____ was a problem in all groups, especially blacks who also suffered from a lack of riboflavin. Vitamin _____ was a concern among teenagers and Spanish Americans.

32. There was a high prevalence of _____ deficiencies.

33. Sugar intake was _____ in most groups, linked with dental _____.

34. Groups needing help with nutrition included obese people, _____, Spanish and Mexican Americans, _____, and low-income families.

Nutrition Canada

35. Canada conducted a major survey of its people in the early _____ including _____ people of all ages and economic levels.

36. Their results were _____ (very similar to/completely different from) those of the Ten State Survey.

The HANES and the Nationwide Food Consumption Survey

37. HANES stands for Health and Nutrition _____ Survey and it avoided the _____ of the earlier survey which was said to oversample vulnerable groups. It involved _____ people at 65 different sites.

38. Nutrient deficiencies were found only for protein, _____, vitamin _____, and iron.

39. HANES II was conducted in _____ to determine whether the physical condition of the subjects studied reflected the _____ intakes found.

40. Not everyone with low intakes of a nutrient had _____ lab values.

41. The HANES researchers observed that there is a continuing trend toward higher amounts of _____ _____ among Americans.

42. Improved protein intakes _____ (can/cannot) alter the average height of a population over several generations.

43. Probably _____ deficiency is the most common vitamin deficiency of all, and it has not yet been included in a survey.

44. The Nationwide Food Consumption Survey showed that _____ seemed to be more of a problem then excess kcalorie intake.

45. _____ million people in the United States are now living at below the poverty level.

46. Interesting trends shown by the survey were that most diets were high in _____, _____, and _____.

47. Americans seem to be eating _____ (very similar/very different) foods.

FOOD CHOICES

48. No matter how nutritious a meal is, it cannot be of benefit until it is _____.

Personal Preference, Habit, Tradition

49. Two preferences widely shared are for _____ and _____. This is an instinctive liking and helped promote early peoples' finding and eating lifegiving foods.

50. Another kind of liking is for foods with which you have _____ associations.

51. Custom sometimes masquerades as family _____.

Social Pressure

52. It is considered _____ not to accept food or drink being offered in a social situation.

53. Besides the food, there is also the pressure of social _____.

Availability/Convenience/Economy

54. Technology has made _____ foods available year around.

55. Many aspects of this constant food supply have put a drain on our _____ supply.

56. We should ask ourselves, "How did the production of this food affect the _____?"

Nutritional Value

57. People often do not know on what _____ to choose amoung the many foods available.

DIET PLANNING

58. There is no single "_____ diet."

59. Foods high in complex _____ are grains, seeds, tubers, legumes, etc.

60. Concentrated _____, not to be overused, include sugar, honey, cola beverages, cakes, candies, and so forth.

61. Meats, nuts, butter, margarine and oils are high in _____.

62. Adequate _____ can be obtained from meats, fish, poultry, eggs, cheese, and milk as well as combinations of grains and legumes.

63. Other guidelines include:
    a. controlling _____.
    b. moderate use of _____.
    c. Choose foods with ample amounts of essential _____ and _____.
    d. Be moderate in use of _____.

64. In China adults obtain calcium through the use of _____, _____, and soybean _____ (which is called tofu).

Coping with the New Foods

65. Reading _____ can be helpful in determining whether foods are nutritious.

66. One important question to ask yourself is, "how often do I _____ this food?"

67. If a food is a staple, is it really providing its share of needed _____ in its class?

68. Are the _____ important in relation to the
     nutrition provided?

69. Values and _____ contribute to the total health
     picture.

SUMMING UP

REVIEW TEXT. Continue to do self-study assessment to evaluate
your lifestyle in relation to the goal of obtaining good
nutrition.

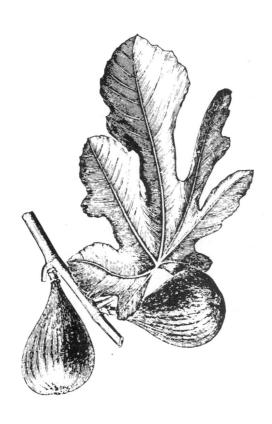

ANSWERS

1. lips
2. assets
    a. taking
    b. measures
    c. examination
    d. analysis
3. history
4. cooking, illnesses
5. recall
6. usual
7. checklist
8. diary
9. RDA
10. guarantee
11. physical, development
12. standards
13. weight
14. skin, tract
15. urine
16. creatinine
17. nutrients
18. protein, kwashiorkor
19. immune
20. cannot
21. is not
22. can
23. can
24. cannot
25. 1/3
26. a. Enrichment
    b. School Lunch
    c. iodine
27. calcium, iron, thiamin, riboflavin, vitamin C
28. 60,000
29. clinical, examinations, measures, case
30. poorer, poor

31. iron, C
32. nutrient
33. high, decay
34. blacks, adolescents
35. 1970's, 19,000
36. very similar to
37. Examination, bias, 20,000
38. calcium, A
39. 1977, nutrient
40. low
41. body fat
42. can
43. folacin
44. inactivity
45. Nineteen
46. fat, sugar, cholesterol
47. very similar
48. eaten
49. sugar, salt
50. happy
51. wisdom
52. rude
53. obligation
54. seasonal
55. energy
56. ecology
57. basis
58. perfect
59. carbohydrates
60. sweets
61. fat
62. protein
63. a. kcalories
     b. sodium
     c. vitamins, minerals
     d. alcohol
64. vegetables, soybeans, curd
65. labels
66. eat
67. nutrients
68. kcalories
69. lifestyle

HIGHLIGHT 12:   THE NEW FOODS AND NUTRITION LABELING

THE NEW FOODS AND NUTRITION LABELING

1. About _____ of all meals are now prepared outside
    the home.

Note to student: Review miniglossary of food types so you
understand the vocabulary used in this highlight.

2. The term "enriched" traditionally refers to four nutrients:
    _____, _____, _____, and
    _____.

3. Fortified refers to the addition of any nutrient to a food
    but sometimes also conveys an _____ of other
    nutrients.

4. The term "nourishing food" and "nutritious foods" are
    _____ (alike/not alike).

Claims and Information on Labels

5. All labels must state:
    a. The common name of the _____.
    b. The _____ and _____ of the manufacturer,
        packer or distributor.
    c. The net _____ in terms of weight, measure, or
        count.
    d. The _____ listed in descending order by weight.

6. Nutrition labeling requirements are imposed on any product
    for which:
    a. _____ claims are made.
    b. For which an _____ claim is made.

7. It is forbidden to say:
   a. That a food is effective as a treatment for a
      _____.
   b. That a balanced diet of ordinary foods cannot supply
      _____ amounts of nutrients.
   c. That the _____ on which food is grown may be
      responsible for deficiencies.
   d. That storage, transportation, processing, etc. may
      be responsible for _____ in its quality.
   e. That a food has particular dietary qualities when such
      _____ have not been shown to be significant.
   f. That a _____ vitamin is superior to a
      _____ - vitamin.

8. When nutrition information is included it must conform to
   the following format:
   a. Serving or _____ size.
   b. Servings or portions per _____.
   c. _____ content per serving.
   d. Protein _____ per serving.
   e. Carbohydrate grams per _____.
   f. Fat _____ per serving.
   g. Protein, vitamins, and minerals as percentages of the
      U.S. RDA. It must provide at least _____ percent
      of that nutrient in a serving before a claim can
      be made.

The U.S. RDA

9. The U.S. RDA was derived mostly from the _____
   tables of _____ to set standards for labeling.

10. There is one recommended amount for each nutrient except
    for _____.

11. Four nutrients that did not appear in the 1968 RDA tables
    were biotin, pantothenic acid, _____ and
    _____. Tentative U.S. RDAs were set for them then
    that have not been changed even though RDAs have now been
    set.

12. Any food claiming to be "low calorie" must contain no more
    than _____ kcalories per serving. Any food calling
    itself a "reduced calorie" food must be at least a
    _____ lower in kcalories than the food it most
    closely resembles and must be labeled. Furthermore,
    wherever additives are listed on labels, their
    _____ must be stated.

HIGHLIGHT 12: THE NEW FOODS AND NUTRITION LABELING

Nutrients in Convenience Foods

13. There are "nutritional _____ quidelines" for the nutrient contents of many kinds of convenience foods. If a product complies with these guidelines it may carry on its label the statement that it "provides nutrients in _____ appropriate for this class of food as determined by the U.S. government."

14. Foods meeting these guidelines must have a certain _____ nutrient level for each _____ kcalories.

15. Standards of Identity exist for common foods that at one time were prepared at _____ and the basic recipe was well understood.

Imitation Food

16. If a food is an imitation of a _____ food, this fact must be stated on the label.

17. Some imitation foods may now be better than traditional foods so the regulation was changed to require the word "_____" only if the product was nutritionally inferior to the food imitated.

18. Nutritional inferiority is defined as a reduction in vitamin, mineral or protein content that amounts to_____ percent or more of the U.S. RDA.

Misleading Labels

19. Misleading claims can be made just by choosing comparisons that are favorable to the manufacturer and probably not well enough understood by the average consummer to know the difference.

Sugar and Salt

20. Consumers want to know the amount of sugar and _____ in foods.

21. Food producers do not want the _____ to put them at an unfair disadvantage.

22. Definitions need to be agreed upon such as how to define
     what is to be called sugar and how it is to be
     _____. If it is listed in grams per _____ it
     will appear differently than stated as a _____.

23. Should salt be listed as salt or _____? Should only
     added salt be listed, or what occurs naturally in the food?

24. Many companies are voluntarily listing sodium in _____
     per serving.

25. Regulations also define listings such as "sodium
     _____," "low sodium, "reduced sodium," and moderately
     low sodium" on labels. Proposed regulations also provide
     for product _____ statements.

26. If the term "unsalted," "without salt added," and "no salt
     added" are used, _____ content also must be listed.

27. FDA also recommends that potassium _____ be listed
     in nutrition labeling.

28. Sugar and salt _____ (are/are not) additives.

29. The law requires that companies making alcoholic beverages
     should list their ingredients on labels, but they
     _____. (See To Explore Further for answer.)

ANSWERS

1. one-half
2. iron, thiamin, riboflavin, niacin
3. emptiness
4. not alike
5. a. product
    b. name, address
    c. contents
    d. ingredients
6. a. nutrition
    b. advertising
7. a. disease
    b. adequate
    c. soil
    d. deficiencies
    e. qualities
    e. natural, synthetic
8. a. portion
    b. container
    c. Kcalorie
    d. grams
    e. serving
    f. grams
    g. ten
9. RDA, 1968
10. protein
11. copper, zinc
12. 40, third, purpose
13. quality, amounts
14. minimum, 100
15. home
16. traditional
17. imitation
18. ten
19. given statement
20. salt
21. labels

22.   listed, serving, percentage
23.   sodium
24.   grams
25.   free, comparative
26.   sodium
27.   content
28.   are
29.   don't

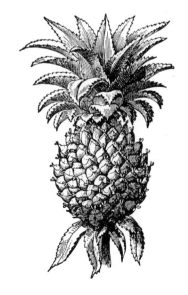

SELF TEST

1. Four techniques to assess nutrition status of an individual
    are used. They include <u>all but one</u> of the following:
    a. use of the Basic Four food groups.
    b. lab tests.
    c. physical examination.
    d. anthropometric measures.
    e. history taking.

2. Means of obtaining food intake data include <u>all but one</u> of
    the following:
    a. use of exchange lists.
    b. 24-hour recall.
    c. food diary.
    d. food frequency record.

3. Anthropometrics involve:
    a. lab tests.
    b. chemical tests.
    c. physical measurements.
    d. none of the above
    e. all of the above

4. A test of immune competence is:
    a. antigen skin testing.
    b. immunology.
    c. serum allergy.
    d. red blood cell count.

5. Computer diet analysis is most severely limited in validity
    because of:
    a. poorly written programs.
    b. incompetent and poorly trained operators.
    c. inaccurate food composition data.
    d. slow computers.

6. Hair analysis is becoming a very important tool in
    analyzing nutrition status of individuals:
    a. true
    b. false

7. The Enrichment Act provides that refined bread and grain
    products should have added:

    a. iron, thiamin, riboflavin, and niacin.
    b. niacin, riboflavin and thiamin.
    c. thaimin, folacin, riboflavin and niacin.

8. A school lunch is supposed to provide:
    a. one-sixth of the RDA for all of the nutrients.
    b. one-third of the RDA for all the nutrients.
    c. one-half of the RDA for all the nutrients.
    d. none of the above

9. Data from nutrition status surveys prior to 1970 revealed
    widespread deficiencies of:
    a. vitamin B_6 and folacin.
    b. iron, zinc, magnesium, and thiamin.
    c. vitamins A, C, and folacin.
    d. all of the above
    e. none of the above

10. Low-income people had nutrition that was _____ than
    that of people in other groups:
    a. better
    b. worse
    c. the same

11. The Ten State Survey showed that:
    a. U.S. citizens eat very well.
    b. only the poorer groups show any deficiencies.
    c. people do not eat as well as might be expected
        in such a prosperous nation.
    d. protein is a problem for pregnant and lactating women.
    e. c and d

12. The results of Canada's survey, compared to the U.S.
    surveys were:
    a. much the same.
    b. much better.
    c. much poorer.

13. Obese people were shown by the Nationwide Food Consumption Survey to:

    a. overeat kcalories by 10-20 percent.
    b. have a quite modest kcalorie intake.
    c. be extraordinarily inactive.
    d. a and c
    e. b and c

14. The Nationwide Food Consumption Survey also showed that:
    a. regional and ethnic differences made food consumption vary widely.
    b. Americans were, for the most part, eating from a common table.
    c. the Four Food Group plan was very successful in offering guidelines for food choices.
    d. none of the above
    e. all of the above

15. In making food choices, it was found that nutritional value ("I thought they were good for me") was the most important guideline that people considered.
    a. true
    b. false

16. A common taste that all people seem to share is the taste for:
    a. sweet and sour.
    b. bitter and salty.
    c. sugar and salt.
    d. all of the above

17. If you find yourself eating ice cream and cake at a birthday party, even though you are on a diet, you may be yielding to:
    a. weak willpower.
    b. social pressure.
    c. your inborn taste for sweets.
    d. a and c
    e. a, b, and c

18. Factors to consider in choosing foods in the future must
    include:
    a.   energy cost.
    b.   impact on the ecology.
    c.   nutrient density.
    d.   a and c
    e.   a, b, and c

19. The "perfect diet" has been formulated by nutritionists and
    is taught as:
    a.   The Four Food Group plan.
    b.   the Exchange food system.
    c.   the Prudent Diet.
    d.   none of the above
    e.   all of the above

20. Meat is a source of:
    a.   protein.
    b.   fat.
    c.   carbohydrate.
    d.   a and b

21. Soybean curd is a rich source of:
    a.   protein.
    b.   calcium.
    c.   kcalories.
    d.   a and b
    e.   a, b, and c

ANSWERS

1. a
2. a
3. c
4. a
5. c
6. b
7. a
8. b
9. e
10. b
11. e
12. a
13. e
14. b
15. b
16. c
17. e
18. e
19. d
20. d
21. d

"EAT-IN" WITHOUT COOKING...

You can have nourishing meals or snacks without a stove, a refrigerator or much money. These same ideas can be used when you travel.

For Breakfast

Orange slices or sections, grapefruit or Vitamin C crystals
    dissolved in water.
Ready-to-eat cereals with milk.
Melba toast with peanut butter or cheese.
Milk to drink (fresh, evaporated or non-fat powdered milk).
Instant tea, coffee or cocoa (if tap water is hot).
(Use evaporated milk or double-strength reconstituted dry milk
in tea or coffee if you use it).

For Lunch or Supper

Salad plate of: tuna or cold cuts, tomato slices or wedges, green pepper rings or carrot strips. Add canned vegetables of some kind--carrots, beets, corn, peas or green beans.

Sandwich--cold cuts or canned meat and cheese with some fruit and vegetables.

Bread or crackers with peanut butter.
Fruit in season or canned fruit.
Milk, tea or coffee.

For Snacks

Fruit and cheese
Crackers and cheese
Crackers and milk

Cereal and milk
Crackers and peanut butter
Roasted peanuts

RECIPES YOU CAN TRY...

These foods need no refrigeration before opening:

Canned meat: tuna, salmon, sardines.
Canned vegetables: peas, beans, beets, corn, sweet potatoes,
                    diced carrots, spinach, etc.
Canned fruits: applesauce, apricots, peaches, pears, pineapple,
                plums, fruit cocktail.
Dried fruits and nuts: raisins, prunes, peanuts, etc.
Fresh fruits with skins: apples, bananas, grapefruit, grapes,
                          oranges, pears, tangerines, etc.
Non-fat or low-fat dry milk.
Evaporated milk (use in 1-2 days once opened.)
Peanut butter.
Jelly, jam, honey or molasses.
Small chunks of cheese tightly wrapped in foil.
Tea bags, instant tea, coffee or cocoa.
Bread wrapped in its original wrapping.
Ready-to-eat cereals.
Oatmeal cookies or crackers.

Tips to Remember about Food Storage

...keep food in the driest and coolest spot in room.
...keep all food covered at all times.
...Open food boxes or cans carefully so that you can close
   them tightly after each use.
...Wrap bread, cookies or crackers in plastic bags and keep
   them in tight containers.
...Empty opened packages of sugar, dried fruits or nuts into
   screw-top jars or airtight tin cans.

Basic Equipment You Need to Have

Cups and/or glasses   Small bowls
Can opener   Paper plates
Knives, forks, spoons   Paring knife
Heating coil*

    *This costs about $2-$5. You can plug it into an electric
outlet, immerse the coil in a cup of water and boil the water.
You can also make boiled eggs or warm soup with it.

    A hot plate and a small toaster-oven are helpful appliances
that add much more variety to your meals. In might even be
possible to have an inexpensive foam ice chest to provide a
cooler storage place.

CHAPTER 13
Mother and Infant

YOU WILL LEARN...

1. How a mother's poor nutrition in early pregnancy can even affect her grandchild.

2. The anatomy of the reproductive system.

3. The importance of nutrition during critical periods of fetal growth.

4. How much weight a pregnant woman should gain.

5. How to have a healthy pregnancy and avoid problems.

6. The preparation necessary for breastfeeding.

7. What pregnant and lactating mothers need to eat.

8. The information necessary to nourish a baby.

9. How to get a child to develop good eating habits.

10. Information helpful in deciding whether or not you would want to breastfeed your baby.

MOTHER AND INFANT

PREGNANCY: THE IMPACT OF NUTRITION ON THE FUTURE

1. The only way nutrients can reach the developing infant in
    the uterus is through the mother's _____.

2. Nutrition status before pregnancy affects the size of the
    _____.

3. If you start eating a good diet as soon as you know you are
    pregnant, you still can't make up for pre-pregnancy
    _____.

4. Poor nutrition of a woman during early pregnancy can even
    affect the health of her _____, even after that
    child has become an adult.

Critical Periods

5. A potential mother should take no _____ at all, not even
    _____.

6. A period during development in which certain events may
    occur that will have irreversible consequence is called a
    _____ _____.

7. A critical period is usually a period of _____
    _____ in a body organ.

8. A developing infant is called an _____ or zygote
    before the second week, an _____ during the second to
    eighth week after conception, and then a _____
    until birth.

9. During the first year after birth, the _____ doubles in
    weight, and after that grows another 20 percent.

10. The systems first to reach maturity are the _____ and central _____ system.

11. Each organ needs the growth nutrients most during its own _____ growth period.

12. An increase in cell <u>number</u> is called _____.

13. An increase in cell <u>size</u> is called _____.

14. There can be simultaneous hyperplasia and _____.

15. Malnutrition in the prenatal and early postnatal periods also affects learning _____ and _____.

16. Severe mental retardation can be due to _____ deficiency during pregnancy.

Fetal Growth

17. The fetal period is the last _____ months of pregnancy.

18. The normal weight gain of mother and child during pregnancy is about _____ to _____ pounds.

19. It is normal for a pregnant woman to seem _____, retain water, and have a changed blood sugar reading.

20. Laboratory tests may show that values for protein, iron, folacin, and other nutrients are lowered, while values for _____ and fat-soluble vitamins may rise.

Nutrient Needs

21. An increase in kcalories is needed only in the last half of pregnancy, and it could be as little as a _____ percent increase though some individuals may need more.

22. However, individual nutrients need to be increased considerably such as iron, _____, folacin, calcium, phosphorus, and magnesium.

23. The body partially makes up for the increased need of iron by _____ it.

Eating Pattern and Weight Gain

24. In the Four Food Group System, recommended servings increase in everything except _____ and _____. There is no place in the diet for _____kcalorie foods since the principle of nutrient density is all-important.

25. Very often, a low-birthweight baby is a _____ baby.

26. A baby weighing less than _____ pounds is considered a low-birthweight baby even if it is full term. This occurs in the United States in about one in every _____ infants born and about 1/4 of them die within the first month of life.

27. About _____ of all cases of mental retardation worldwide could be eliminated by improved maternal and infant care programs.

Practices to Avoid

28. Having a healthy baby requires knowledge and discipline. Harmful influences during pregnancy include drugs, dieting, _____ , protein deprivation, and alcohol.

29. Brain damage and irreversible mental and physical retardation caused by a mother who consumed excess alcohol during pregnancy is called fetal _____ _____.

30. Use of caffeine, sugar, and saccharin should be _____.

Troubleshooting

31. A cluster of symptoms seen in pregnancy including edema, hypertension, and kidney complications is called _____.

32. Salt restriction is a/an _____ (wise/unwise) practice for a healthy woman to follow during pregnancy.

33. Iron and _____ supplements are often prescribed to help prevent the two common anemias of pregnancy.

34. Other important nutritional pointers for pregnancy are to include adequate vitamin B_6, a high-fiber diet, and after the fifth month, _____, either from water or a supplement.

35. A craving for clay, ice, cornstarch, or other nonnutritious substances is called _____ and reflects a real need for iron or _____, neither of which are present in the substances craved. This is called non-adaptive behavior.

Preparing for Breastfeeding

36. Preparing for breastfeeding could include:
    a. reading books, talking to successful mothers who have nursed, or other supportive advisors.
    b. acquiring nursing bras.
    c. "toughening" the _____.

BREASTFEEDING

37. Adequate _____ of the mother makes a highly significant contribution to successful _____.

Nutrient Needs

38. The energy allowance for a lactating woman is a generous _____ kcalories per day above her ordinary need. The RDA table suggests that _____ kcalories come from added food, and the rest from the stores of fat accumulated during pregnancy.

39. Needs of calcium, phosphorus, magnesium, and _____ continue to be high. Iron and _____ needs decrease from the level necessary during pregnancy.

Eating Pattern

40. A new mother needs to drink plenty of _____. If she can't drink cow's milk, nutritionally similar substitutes such as cheese, _____ milk, and greens would be good choices.

41. The effect of nutrition deprivation of the mother is to reduce the _____, not the quality, of her milk.

42. The nutrient concentration of breast milk _____
     (does/does not) appear to remain relatively constant.

Advantages of Breastfeeding

43. The premilk substance produced by the breasts is called
     _____. It contains many antibodies that pass on
     the mother's immunities to the child.

44. Milk is not a good source of vitamin _____, but this
     vitamin is provided adequately for the human infant in
     breast milk.

45. The chief protein in human breast milk is called
     _____. The chief protein of cow's milk is
     _____.

46. Breast milk is _____ (low/high) in sodium.

47. In breast milk, _____% of the iron is absorbed,
     compared with only _____% from fortified formula.
     Zinc is also better absorbed from breast milk because of an
     important zinc-binding protein.

48. Another factor in breast milk that is important is
     _____, which binds iron and keeps it from
     supporting the growth of infectious bacteria in the infant.

49. Breast milk also contains _____, and also
     contains a factor that favors the growth of
     "_____" bacteria, called the _____
     factor.

50. There are other important advantages to breast feeding that
     are being researched including important _____,
     hormones, and other compounds that are beneficial to the
     infant as well as the mother.

51. A woman who wants to breastfeed can derive justification
     and _____ from all of these advantages.

Advantages of Formula feeding

52. Cow's milk is significantly higher in protein,
     _____, and phosphorus.

53. To praise breastfeeding out of proportion or without
     qualification can make a mother who bottle fed her baby
     feel _____ or angry.

54. Breastfeeding at first and weaning the infant after one to six months is a good _____ for many.

55. It is important that the baby be weaned onto _____ and not just plain milk.

When Breastfeeding is Preferred

56. When the infant is premature, if the family is _____, or if other factors are against the baby, then _____ is the preferred choice.

57. Aseptic _____ means working in a sterile fashion, keeping an area free of bacteria and other contamination.

58. Breast milk _____ (can be/cannot be) satisfactorily frozen for up to six months.

How to breastfeed

59. After birth, the baby should be nursed within the first _____ minutes to get breastfeeding off to a good start.

60. The formation of a physical and emotional tie between mother and infant is called _____. This also occurs in the first _____ minutes after birth.

61. Beginning at the first feeding the mother should learn how to _____ and make both herself and the baby comfortable.

62. The regulator of the human milk supply is a _____ called prolactin. The infant's sucking action stimulates the release of this hormone.

63. The _____ reflex makes a newborn turn towards whichever cheek is touched and search for the nipple.

64. The let-down or _____-ejection reflex makes the milk flow when the mother perceives the need. The hormone that initiates let-down is _____. The let-down reflex forces milk to the front of the breast.

65. The _____ reflex, occuring later, draws milk from the milk-producing glands at the back. Hindmilk is _____ in fat than foremilk.

66.   The baby can suck _____ the milk from the breast within
      two minutes and 80-90 percent of it within _____
      minutes. After _____ minutes the baby can be given
      the other breast to finish nursing.

67.   Demand feedings, no fewer than _____ per day, are most
      likely to promote optimal milk production and infant
      growth. The first two weeks a mother might even nurse her
      baby _____ times a day to establish successful
      lactation.

Troubleshooting

68.   Sore nipples should be treated _____.

69.   Overfilling of the breasts with milk is called
      _____.

70.   A lump can occur in the breast from an undrained
      _____.

71.   Infants fed sweetened water in the first few months may
      tend to have a greater _____ for sweets later in
      infancy.

72.   Infection of a breast is best managed by _____ to
      breastfeed. This _____ (will/will not) infect the
      infant.

73.   The hormones in _____ contraceptives can _____
      lactation.

74.   A baby's small bowel movements indicate that it
      _____ (is/is not) getting enough milk.

WHEN NOT TO BREASTFEED

75.   A serious communicable disease may cause a mother to be
      separated from her baby. Drug _____, alcohol
      _____ and other problems may prevent safe
      breastfeeding.

76.   Most prescription drugs, moderate alcohol use, smoking, and
      _____ drinking during breastfeeding
      apparently do not affect the baby. The eating of foods
      such as garlic and spices may affect the taste of milk.

77. DDT has been reported in the milk of mothers at higher concentrations than are allowed in _____ milk, and in some cases PCBs have contaminated breast milk as well.

How to Feed Formula

78. AAP stands for the American Association of _____. Any formula meeting the AAP _____ should be satisfactory for a normal baby.

79. Megadoses of vitamin B_6 may suppress _____, as does an injection of estrogen given by the physician.

80. Formula can be offered warm or _____. Whole milk should not be used. A mother mixing or bottling her own formula must use sanitary techniques.

81. Close _____ during feeding is important. Next comes "_____ the baby."

82. Babies should not be allowed to sleep with a _____ because of the danger of tooth decay.

VITAMIN-MINERAL SUPPLEMENTS FOR THE INFANT

83. Only three nutrients may have to be used to supplement breast milk. They are vitamin _____, fluoride, and possibly _____.

84. Formula-fed babies need vitamins _____, C, and _____ as well as fluoride. The makeup of various formulas differ so the contents need to be checked.

NUTRITION OF THE INFANT

85. The baby grows faster during the first _____ than ever again. Growth directly reflects _____ well-being. The birthweight doubles in _____ months.

86. Infants can digest lactose immediately but do not produce amylase until about three months of age, and so cannot digest _____ until then.

87. A baby's energy needs are _____ (high/low).

333

CHAPTER 13: MOTHER AND INFANT

Nutrient Needs

88. The nutrient hardest to provide for infants is
_____.

First Foods

89. A breastfed baby can wait until about _____ months
before receiving solid food, but not longer.

90. Introducing foods too early can cause _____.

91. A term used to mean supplemental or weaning foods is
_____.

92. Nutrients needed early by the formula-fed baby are
_____ and vitamin _____.

93. To help establish beneficial feeding habits for later, it
is now recommended to introduce vegetables _____ and
fruits _____.

94. Solid foods introduced at bedtime _____ (will/will
not) help the baby sleep through the night.

95. New foods should be introduced singly so that
_____ can be detected. Allergies may not show up
until several days after the offending food is eaten.

96. If you want to "blenderize" table food for the baby, it is
necessary to omit _____ in the preparation. Babies
should never be fed _____ vegetables to protect
against _____ contamination.

97. Home prepared carrots, beets, and spinach may contain
_____.

98. Honey should never be fed to infants because of the risk of
_____.

99. A one-year old should be sitting at the table and eating
the _____ everyone else eats.

Looking Ahead

100. The first year of a baby's life is the time to lay the
foundation for future _____.

101. _____ obesity should be avoided. Psychological and nutrition factors both must be considered to prevent the wrong habits from being formed.

102. So far, the "prudent diet" seems to have done infants no _____.

Mealtimes

103. The wise parent of a one-year-old offers _____ and _____ together. Both promote growth. Better brain development occurs with environmental stimulation as well as nutrients.

104. It is important for a child to develop a sense of _____ that will provide the foundation for later confidence and effectiveness as an individual.

105. A child's impulses, if consistently _____, can turn to shame and self-doubt.

SUMMING UP

Review text if necessary

ANSWERS

1.   bloodstream
2.   placenta
3.   malnutrition
4.   grandchild
5.   drugs, aspirin
6.   critical period
7.   cell division
8.   ovum, embryo, fetus
9.   brain
10. brain, nervous
11. intensive
12. hyperplasia
13. hypertrophy
14. hypertrophy
15. ability, behavior
16. protein
17. seven
18. 25, 30
19. anemic
20. cholesterol
21. 15%
22. protein
23. conserving
24. breads, cereals, empty
25. malnourished
26. 5-1/2, 15
27. half
28. smoking
29. alcohol syndrome
30. moderate
31. toxemia
32. unwise
33. folacin
34. fluoride
35. pica, zinc
36. nipples

37.   nutrition, lactation
38.   750, 500
39.   protein, folacin
40.   milk, soy
41.   quantity
42.   does
43.   colostrum
44.   C
45.   lactalbumin, casein
46.   low
47.   49, 4
48.   lactoferrin,
49.   antibodies, friendly, bifidus.
50.   enzymes
51.   satisfaction
52.   calcium
53.   guilty
54.   compromise
55.   formula
56.   poor, breastfeeding
57.   technique
58.   can be
59.   30
60.   bonding, 30
61.   relax
62.   hormone
63.   rooting
64.   milk, oxytocin
65.   draught, higher
66.   half, four, ten
67.   six, twelve
68.   kindly
69.   engorgement
70.   sinus
71.   preference
72.   continuing, will not
73.   oral, suppress
74.   is
75.   addiction, abuse
76.   coffee
77.   cow's
78.   Pediatrics, standards
79.   lactation
80.   cold
81.   contact, burping
82.   bottle
83.   D, iron
84.   A, iron
85.   year, nutrition, four

86.   starch
87.   high
88.   iron
89.   six
90.   allergies
91.   beikost
92.   iron, C
93.   first, later
94.   will not
95.   allergies
96.   salt, canned, lead
97.   nitrates
98.   botulism
99.   food
100. health
101. Infant
102. harm
103. love, food
104. autonomy
105. denied

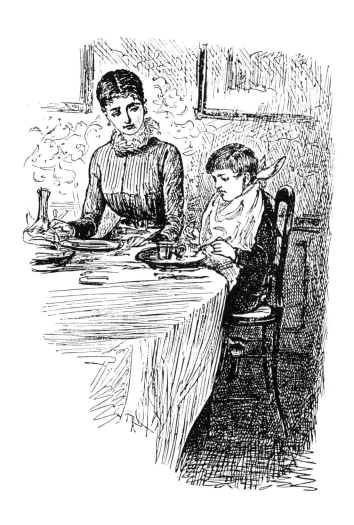

CHAPTER 13: MOTHER AND INFANT

SELF TEST

1. Records maintained during hard times in World War II showed that more birth defects and stillbirths were caused by poor diet before pregnancy than during pregnancy.
   a. true.
   b. false.

2. A critical period is the:
   a. first two weeks after conception.
   b. twenty-four hours after taking a drug that could affect intrauterine events.
   c. a period of cell division in a body organ.
   d. a time of organ growth.

3. The growth stage when cells are dividing rapidly (increasing cell number) is know as:
   a. hypertrophy.
   b. hyperplasia.
   c. the postnatal period.
   d. colostrum.

4. Nutrients and oxygen travel to the developing fetus via:
   a. the amniotic sac.
   b. its lungs.
   c. its intestines.
   d. the placenta.

5. A healthy weight gain during pregnancy is about:
   a. 12-15 pounds.
   b. 25-30 pounds.
   c. 20 pounds.
   d. 35 pounds.

6. A woman weighing 120 lb should have a minimum calorie
    intake while pregnant of about:
    a. 1,000 to 1,500 kcalories per day.
    b. 2,000 to 2,200 kcalories per day.
    c. 2,500 to 3,000 kcalories per day.

7. The pregnant woman has an outstandingly high need for
    _____ as compared to the non-pregnant woman.
    a. kcalories
    b. water
    c. folacin
    d. potassium

8. Among other things, a pregnant woman needs:
    a. 4 glasses of milk a day.
    b. 6 servings of vitamin C-rich foods a day.
    c. 2 servings of breads and cereals a day.
    d. all of the above

9. A low birthweight baby weighs:
    a. less than 1,000 grams at birth.
    b. less than 2,000 grams at birth.
    c. less than 2,500 grams at birth.
    d. less than 5,000 grams at birth.

10. A maternal practice that may be harmful to an unborn child
    is:
    a. smoking.
    b. protein deprivation.
    c. use of a low-carbohydrate diet.
    d. drinking alcohol.
    e. all of the above

11. Toxemia during pregnancy may be due to:
    a. excessive sodium intakes.
    b. excessive water intakes.
    c. a low-protein diet.
    d. a high-protein diet.

12. An unnatural taste for clay, ice, cornstarch and other
    non-nutritious substances is:
    a. a need for support, understanding, and love.
    b. called pica.
    c. a psychological craving.
    d. an adaptive behavior for needed nutrients.

13.   The factor in breast milk that establishes friendly
      bacteria in the intestinal tract is called:
      a.   bifidus.
      b.   colostrum.
      c.   lactalbumin.
      d.   casein.
      e.   lactoferrin.

14.   The predominant protein in human milk is:
      a.   lactalbumin.
      b.   casein.
      c.   lactoferrin.
      d.   colostrum.

15.   Two nutrients for which supplementation is recommended to
      meet the increased requirements for pregnancy are:
      a.   iron and folacin.
      b.   iron and calcium.
      c.   zinc and folacin.
      d.   iodine and calcium.

16.   The mineral that is most related to the expansion of blood
      volume in pregnancy and therefore is of concern in toxemia
      of pregnancy is:
      a.   magnesium.
      b.   iron.
      c.   sodium
      d.   calcium.

17.   Which of the following does not increase a pregnant
      woman's chances of having a low birthweight infant?
      a.   Consuming a high sodium diet during pregnancy.
      b.   Having the first baby before age 17 or after age 35.
      c.   Smoking cigarettes.
      d.   Failing to gain the recommended amount of weight while
           pregnant.

18.   Which of the following statements about breast milk is
      true?
      a.   It is lower in protein than cow's milk.
      b.   It is generally less nourishing for infants than baby
           formula.
      c.   It is more likely to cause allergy than formula.
      d.   all of the above

19.   Because of the dangers of obesity, an overweight woman
      should try to gain little or no weight during pregnancy.
      a.   true.
      b.   false.

20. If a mother finds she cannot breastfeed, the baby can be weaned onto:
    a. whole milk.
    b. low-fat milk.
    c. formula.

21. Bonding between mother and infant usually takes place:
    a. immediately after birth.
    b. within the first three months after birth.
    c. in the first 45 minutes after birth.
    d. all of the above

22. It is not possible to become pregnant while breastfeeding.
    a. true
    b. false

23. If a baby is getting enought breastmilk it tends to have:
    a. large bowel movements
    b. small bowel movements.

24. Breastmilk is high in vitamin D.
    a. true
    b. false

25. When the baby is eating solid foods, which should be introduced first?
    a. Fruits
    b. Vegetables

26.- 29. Matching - Feeding the infant. Match the stage or appropriate action with the infant's age.
    (a) one day old   (b) 3 months old   (c) 4-6 months old
    (d) one year old

_____ 26. Unable to digest starch until this age.
_____ 27. A good age to introduce solids.
_____ 28. Skim milk should not be used until this age.
_____ 29. A breastfed baby receives colostrum at this age.

30. Introducing solids to an infant will help it sleep through the night.
    a. true
    b. false

31. If a baby is thirsty, you should give it a bottle of:
    a. fruit juice.
    b. sweetened water.
    c. formula.
    d. water.

32. Growth is much more rapid during the second year of life than during the first year.
    a. true
    b. false

33. In the United States, one out of every _____ babies is born to a mother under 19 years of age.
    a. 3
    b. 4
    c. 5
    d. 10

34. An example of an inborn error is:
    a. lactose intolerance.
    b. low birth weight.
    c. fetal alcohol syndrome.
    d. all of the above

ANSWERS

1.   a
2.   c
3.   b
4.   d
5.   b
6.   b
7.   c
8.   a
9.   c
10.   e
11.   c
12.   b
13.   a
14.   a
15.   a
16.   c
17.   a
18.   a
19.   b
20.   c
21.   c
22.   b
23.   b
24.   b
25.   b
26.   b
27.   c
28.   d
29.   a
30.   b
31.   d
32.   b
33.   c
34.   c

MAKING YOUR OWN BABY FOOD...

TIPS FOR MAKING YOUR OWN BABY FOOD:

Homemade baby foods are an economical and easy way to feed your baby providing you use high-quality ingredients; do not add unnecessary extras, such as salt, monosodium glutamate, sugar, or other sweeteners to them; and prepare them with the utmost cleanliness--clean hands, clean kitchen, clean utensils, clean food and clean storage containers. Homemade baby foods offer the advantage of using the same foods prepared for the family meals, which can be separated before salt and other seasonings are added and pureed for the baby to eat right away--or frozen for later use.

GUIDELINES FOR PREPARING BABY FOOD:

....Be sure everything is clean, use fresh foods. Do not use regular canned fruits and vegetables because of the potentially high lead content of the cans.

....Be sure to remove all skin, pits, and seeds from fruits and vegetables and excess fat and gristle--and the bones--from meat and poultry.

....Add a small amount of water to foods and cook just until tender. Save unsalted cooking liquid for pureeing.

....Place the cooked food into a baby food grinder, blender, food processor, or mash with a fork through a strainer. Add cooking liquid, broth, milk, or water to blend the food to baby food consistency.

....Never put the same spoon back into the food if you taste the baby food...it can cause the food to spoil and can spread any germs from your mouth to the baby.

HOW TO STORE HOMEMADE BABY FOODS:

Homemade strained baby foods can be stored in ice cube trays or individual ice cube containers. After the food is frozen, the cubes can be popped out and stored in tightly sealed plastic bags in the freezer. To thaw, place frozen cube in a custard cup or other heatproof dish and set the dish in hot water. Be sure to date and label all frozen baby foods and try to use within one month so they will not lose their nutritional value.

....Avoid freezing foods that have been stored in the refrigerator even for one day.

....Avoid refreezing foods that have been previously frozen.

....Avoid storing home-prepared baby foods in the refrigerator for longer than two days.

IMPORTANT THINGS TO KNOW ABOUT USING COMMERCIAL BABY FOODS.

....Always wash the baby food jar before opening.

....When you open the jar, listen for a "pop" sound. This will tell you that the protective seal has not been previously broken (and that bacteria have not contaminated the food).

....Put the amount of food that you think the baby will eat in a clean dish, replace the jar lid, and refrigerate the remaining food in the jar immediately...the leftover food should be used within two days.

....Do not feed directly from the jar unless you know that the baby will eat the entire contents of the jar.

....Throw away any food remaining in the dish after the baby is finished eating.

....Read the ingredient labels carefully. Look for foods that don't list any added starch, sugar or salt. Steer clear of foods that list water first.

....Meats are probably your best buy. They may contain added salt but generally no starch or sugar.

....Avoid the desserts. They tend to have a lot of added ingredients and are unnecessary in baby's diet

RECIPES YOU CAN TRY...

TEETHING BISCUITS

1 beaten egg yolk
1 tsp vanilla
2 tbsp honey
2 tbsp molasses
2 tbsp salad oil

3/4 cup whole wheat flour
1 tbsp wheat germ
1 tbsp soy flour
1-1/2 tbsp nonfat dry
   milk powder

Blend egg yolk, vanilla, honey, molasses and oil, and mix in the blended whole wheat and soy flours, wheat germ and nonfat dry milk powder. Roll out dough very thinly, 1/8 to 1/4 inch. Cut in baby-finger-length rectangles. Bake at 350 degrees F. on ungreased cookie sheet for 15 minutes. Remove from sheet and cool thoroughly on cake racks. Store in tightly covered container.

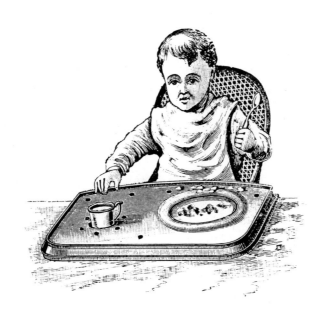

CHAPTER 14
Child and Teen

YOU WILL LEARN...

1. How observations made on populations during times of change in their food supplies reveal important information about the maturity, stature, and development of the people.

2. How early childhood nutrition affects the adult.

3. The way schools participate in pre-adolescent nutrition.

4. The influence of television on food choices.

5. What might be done to alter diets to prevent diseases and disorders of adulthood.

6. Factors influencing teen eating patterns, and possible solutions.

7. Important information to help understand unfortunate disorders known as bulimia and anorexia nervosa.

8. Why teenage pregnancy is so risky to mother and child.

9. How alcohol and drugs affect nutrition and well-being.

10. Why some teenagers develop poor food choices and some possible solutions.

CHILD AND TEEN

1. Optimal nutrition permits development to realize its full
    _____.

SECULAR TRENDS IN NUTRITION

2. Observations made on populations during times of change in
    their food supplies have demonstrated important effects on
    the timing of young people's maturation. These effects,
    measured in years, are know as _____
    _____ in nutrition.

3. The age at which the first menstrual period occurs is
    called _____.

4. All environmental conditions must be ideal for a person to
    reach their full _____ potential.

5. Sometimes it is impossible to know what that potential is
    because we may not have reached it yet. Yet the secular
    trend shows that _____ has now decreased since
    1930 and full height is achieved for males by _____ or
    19.

6. Because of increased _____ intake, the Japanese
    people have steadily increased their height since 1900,
    except when food deprivation was severe.

EARLY CHILDHOOD

7. The growth patterns of girls and boys begin to become
    distinct just before _____, at which time fat
    becomes a larger percentage of total body weight for girls,
    and in boys the lean body mass becomes greater.

Nutrition Needs and Feeding

8. The last period in which parents influence food choices significantly is the _____ period.

9. A serving of food for a child from the basic four food groups is loosely defined as 1 tbsp per year, so at age two a child might eat two tbsp of meat, fruits, and vegetables, and at age four, _____ tbsp of each as one serving.

NUTRITION AT SCHOOL

10. The school lunch is intended to provide a least a _____ of the RDA for each of the nutrients. Unfortunately, children don't always _____ what they are served.

11. Since 1980 different meal patterns have been tried to reduce plate _____.
    a. More foods are offered so children can _____ what is served.
    b. Portion sizes now vary.
    c. Students in the secondary schools can now help _____ menus.
    d. lunches are scheduled at better times for the children's needs.

12. Milk is required as part of the school lunch, but it _____ (does/does not) have to be whole milk.

13. Since 1980, _____cents per child is allocated for nutrition education and _____ (NET).

14. Children growing up today need to _____ about nutrition to become able to make _____ food choices.

Television and Vending Machines

15. An average child sees about _____ commercials per year, of which more than half are for _____ foods.

16. Cola beverages and chocolates contain a great deal of _____ as well as sugar.

17. Experiments have shown that many children _____(would/would not) choose nutritions snacks if they were offered side by side with sugary foods.

CHAPTER 14:   CHILD AND TEEN

Looking Ahead

18. To avoid obesity, children should be trained to "eat
     _____," don't always clean their _____,
     and be _____ physically.

19. The most common nutrition disorder after obesity is
     _____ - _____ _____.

20. The prevention of cardiovascular disease may begin in
     childhood.   It is important to learn to avoid snacks that
     are too high in _____, _____ and
     _____.

21. The Guidelines may help prevent the onset of diabetes
     and_____.   One example of a recommended diet
     is called the _____ diet.

22. Another preventable condition is poor _____ health.

23. Good dental health means:
     a. An adequate _____(especially with respect to
         protein; calcium; vitamins A, C, D;
         and _____).
     b. restricting the supply of _____ foods.
     c. proper use of _____ or dental floss.

Mealtimes with Children

24. Strategies to get children to eat vegetables include:

     a. serving them warm instead of _____, and slightly
         undercooked.
     b. making sure they are a pretty _____.
     c. making sure there are no lumps.
     d. present vegetables with a _____ flavor.
     e. making them easy to eat.
     f. maintaining a relaxed and casual atmosphere.

25. Never make an _____ of food acceptance. Avoid a
     power struggle over which foods to eat.

26. The key word at one year is _____.

27. At two years the word is _____. At four years
     the word is _____.

CHAPTER 14:   CHILD AND TEEN

THE TEEN YEARS

28. Teenagers are not fed; they _____.

Growth and Nutrient Needs.

29. The adolescent growth spurt begins in girls at _____ and peaks at age _____, being completed at about _____.

30. In boys, the growth spurt begins at _____ and peaks at _____, ending about _____.

31. Adolescent girls and boys _____(do/do not) need the same amount of kcalories per day.

32. A girl of 15 who is 5' 7" tall should weigh approximately _____pounds, according to the rule of thumb for teen girls.

Eating Patterns

33. On the average, about a _____ of a teenager's total daily kcalorie intake comes from _____.

34. The nutrients most often not obtained in a teen's snack-type diet plan are vitamin _____ and _____.

35. Teenagers' _____ needs are a special problem, partly because they overconsume milk, and partly because of the low contribution of this mineral made by fast foods.

36. Plant foods high in iron are _____ and whole _____.

ANOREXIA NERVOSA AND BULIMIA

37. An extreme preoccupation with _____ loss by a competitive and perfectionistic teenage girl may be the start of a disorder called _____ nervosa.

38. When the anorexic reaches an absolute minimum body weight she is on the verge of incurring permanent _____ damage and chronic _____ or _____. One in five anorexics die.

39. Anorexia nervosa is a disease of the _____ countries.

40. Periodic binge-eating alternating with intervals of dieting or self-starvation is called _____. Another name for this disorder is _____.

41. Another abuse often followed by the anorexic or bulimic person is _____ abuse.

THE PREGNANT TEENAGE GIRL

42. _____ is common in pregnant teenagers because of inadequate nutrient stores.

43. _____ occurs in about one out of every five girls under the age of 15. Close pregnancies could progress to kidney damage and hypertensive _____ disease.

44. One out of every _____ babies is born to a mother under 19 years of age.

45. Pregnant teenagers need medical attention, nutrition guidance, _____ support, and continued _____.

46. WIC stands for Women's, Infants' and _____ program.

ALCOHOL AND DRUGS

47. Complications to nutrition and health during the teen years can come from such diversified problems as:
    a. use and abuse of _____.
    b. prolonged use of prescription_____.
    c. drug _____ and abuse.
    d. overconsumption of caffeine.
    e. oral _____.
    Many of these things come along at a time when nutrition is most inadequate, and are probably compounded by that fact.

48. If heavy drinkers are identified by ethnic groups it is seen that _____ American youth are in the highest proportion and _____ in the lowest.

49. In college about _____percent of students use alcohol. Among adults in the United States, about 100 million drink, and _____ million are estimated to be alcoholics.

50. Is it true that a beer drinker can never become an alcohol addict? _____ (yes/no).

51. The _____ of the consumer determines whether he or she will become addicted to alcohol.

52. The carbonation in beer _____(inhibits/stimulates) the absorption of alcohol into the intestine.

53. If you are on the Pill, you may need less vitamin _____ and _____ and more_____ vitamins and vitamin C.

54. It is _____ (a good idea/probably not necessary) to take a vitamin supplement when on the Pill.

55. Smoking a marihuana cigarette has an effect on hearing, _____, taste, and _____, and on perceptions of time, _____, and the body; it also produces changes in mental sensations and alterations in the nature of _____ .

56. Even a small amount of marihuana smoking can cause driving performance to _____, reduce the body's _____ response and lower _____ count.

57. Since there are no controls on the content of preparations sold as marihuana, they may be _____.

TEENAGERS FOOD CHOICES

58. When the poor food habits of some teenagers were analyzed, it was found that they often:
     a. think nutrition means eating what you don't like.
     b. have unique eating patterns but feel fine.
     c. are _____ in food.
     d. are not hearing the truth about nutrition.

59. Many teenagers are greatly _____ with their bodies.

60. Nutrient-dense, _____ kcalorie foods favor the development of strong _____ in men and an _____ figure in women.

61. Nutrition educators should _____ what they _____ .

62. Teenagers have the _____ to make their own decisions.

SUMMING UP

Review text as necessary

ANSWERS

1. potential
2. secular trends
3. menarche
4. genetic
5. menarche, 18
6. protein
7. adolescence
8. preadolescent
9. four
10. third, eat
11. waste
      a. choose
      c. plan
12. does not
13. nine, training
14. learn, adaptive
15. 10,000, sugary
16. caffeine
17. would
18. thin, plates, active
19. iron-deficiency anemia
20. fat, sugar, salt
21. cancer, prudent
22. dental
23. a. diet, fluoride
      b. sugary
      c. brushing
24. a. hot
      b. color
      d. mild
25. issue
26. trust
27. autonomy, initiative
28. eat
29. 10-11, 12, 14

30. 12-13, 14, 19
31. do not
32. 125
33. fourth, snacks
34. A, folacin
35. iron
36. legumes, grains
37. weight, anorexia
38. brain, invalidism, death
39. developed
40. bulimia, bulimarexia
41. laxative
42. Sickness
43. Toxemia, heart
44. five
45. emotional, schooling
46. Children's
47. a. alcohol
    b. drugs
    c. use
    e. contraceptives
48. Native, blacks
49. 90, 9
50. no
51. constitution
52. stimulates
53. A, iron, B
54. probably not necessary
55. touch, smell, space, sleep
56. deteriorate, immune, sperm
57. contaminated
58. c. uninterested
59. dissatisfied
60. low, muscles, attractive
61. practice, preach
62. right

SELF TEST

1. When nutrition is seen to affect either the timing or extent of maturity in a large group this is identified as a:
   a. replicated study.
   b. nutri-data study.
   c. secular trend.
   d. nutrition-related trend.

2. The term "menarche" is used to describe:
   a. sexual maturity of males.
   b. sexual maturity of females.
   c. the time when nutrient intake improves.
   d. the age at which the first menstrual period occurs.

3. Since 1900, the Japanese people have steadily increased their height because:
   a. more food is available.
   b. they mated with taller people who had dominant genes.
   c. nutrition education was stressed by the government.
   d. they ate more protein.

4. Just before adolescence the growth patterns of girls and boys are:
   a. the same.
   b. different, in that girls have a larger percentage of fat.
   c. different, in that boys have a larger lean body mass.
   d. different, in that boys start out taller.
   e. b and c

5. If a mother is trying to follow the four food group pattern in feeding her three-year old child, it would be appropriate to serve _____ each, for a serving, of meat, fruits, and vegetables:
    a. two tablespoons
    b. three tablespoons
    c. a half cup
    d. none of the above

6. The school lunch is intended to provide _____ of the day's nutrient needs.
    a. one fourth
    b. one third
    c. one half

7. Experiments have shown that children would not choose nutritious snacks if they were offered side by side with sugary foods.
    a. true
    b. false

8. When the prudent diet was tried on a group of children it:
    a. apparently was not harmful.
    b. was greatly disliked by the test group.
    c. proved later to be less nutritious than a regular diet.
    d. was missing several nutrients.

9. Which idea is not effective in helping children to like vegetables:
    a. serve them warm, not hot.
    b. select those with a bright color and mild flavor.
    c. serve them slightly undercooked and crunchy.
    d. withhold dessert until the plate is clean.

10. Which is most important:
    a. teaching children to make adaptive food choices.
    b. withholding junk food so they do not acquire a taste for it.
    c. rewarding a wise choice with a special treat.

11. An average child who watches television sees more than:
    a. 100 commercials in six months.
    b. 500 in a year.
    c. 5,000 in six months.
    d. 5,000 in a year.

12. A child who is at the age when autonomy was the "key" word
    is probably about:
    a. one year of age.
    b. two years of age.
    c. age three.
    d. age five.

13. A girl of 18 years who is 5'7" tall should weigh
    approximately _____, according to the rule of thumb
    for teen girls.
    a. 128
    b. 125
    c. 130
    d. 123

14. Anorexia nervosa has always been common in developing
    countries, and has only been identified here in the last 25
    years.
    a. true
    b. false

15. A person most likely to suffer from anorexia nervosa could
    probably be described as:
    a. having low self esteem.
    b. being a perfectionist.
    c. coming from a weight-conscious family.
    d. having very strong willpower.
    e. all of the above

16. Victims of anorexia nervosa lose their appetites.
    a. true
    b. false

17. A teenager gets about _____ of the day's kcalories from
    snacks.
    a. one fourth
    b. one third
    c. one half

18. Periodic binge-eating alternating with self-starvation or
    purging is called:
    a. bulimia.
    b. bulimarexia.
    c. anorexia.
    d. a and b

19. Pregnant teenagers are _____ likely to have problem pregnancies than women in their twenties.
    a. more
    b. less

20. Beer drinkers are much less likely to become alcoholics than are drinkers of hard liquor.
    a. true
    b. false

21. The carbonation in beer inhibits the absorption of alcohol into the intestine.
    a. true
    b. false

22. There are valuable nutrients in beer that make an important contribution to the diets of those who do not abuse it.
    a. true
    b. false

23. If you are on the Pill, your nutrition status may be enhanced with respect to:
    a. B vitamins and vitamin C.
    b. vitamin A and iron.
    c. calcium and magnesium.

24. If you are on the Pill, your nutrition status may be worsened with respect to:
    a. B vitamins and vitamin C.
    b. vitamin A and iron.
    c. calcium and magnesium.

25. Smoking marihuana can enhance your driving performance by making your reactions faster.
    a. true
    b. false

26. Teenagers should not be allowed to make their own decisions until they are older and have a greater understanding of important facts that influence their lives.
    a. true
    b. false

ANSWERS

1. c
2. d
3. d
4. e
5. b
6. b
7. b
8. a
9. d
10. a
11. c
12. b
13. a
14. b
15. e
16. b
17. a
18. d
19. a
20. b
21. b
22. b
23. b
24. a
25. b
26. b

RECIPES YOU CAN TRY...

SNACK IDEAS USING LESS SUGAR

Most children, teens and adults tend to lack nutrients from milk, fruits, and vegetables. Why not start there?

A glass of milk, flavored or plain	An orange
Custard or pudding	Raw vegetables
Dried prunes or apricots	Cheese and crackers
A handful of peanuts or other nuts	Leftover chicken
A sandwich, taco, or hamburger	Fruit gelatin
Banana, celery, apple or pear slices with peanut butter	Raisins
	Granola
Fruit juice or frozen fruit juice popsicles	Yogurt
	Hard-cooked egg
Cottage cheese and applesauce	Cheese chunks
Beef jerky	Pizza
Cookies made with enriched or whole wheat flour, dried fruit and/or nuts	Instant soup mixes
	Raisins & Sunflower seeds mixed together

All kinds of dried fruits are good as is, but this makes a good combination if you have access to a food grinder.

DRIED FRUIT TREATS

1 cup raisins
1 cup dried pitted prunes
1 cup dried apricots
powdered sugar or coconut flakes

Put all the fruit through a grinder. Run a few crackers through the grinder after the fruit to clean the grinder and keep from wasting the fruit. Mix the ground fruit and crackers together, shape into small balls and roll in either sugar or coconut flakes. Lay them on waxed paper to get firm.

SPACE STICKS

1 cup graham cracker crumbs
1 cup dry milk powder
2/3 cup honey
1 cup peanut butter, chunk style is great

Combine all the ingredients in a bowl and mix it with your hands. Add more graham cracker crumbs if the mixture is too sticky. Pull off pieces of the mixture and roll it into small logs, 1" to 6" in length, depending on your preference. Wrap each piece in aluminum foil. These may be stored in the refrigerator or on the shelf.

For variation add instant chocolate drink powder, raisins, nuts or coconut. This is also great for stuffing celery stalks.

GELATIN FRUIT SQUARES

Flavored gelatin contains 85% sugar, artificial color and flavoring--and very little nutritive value. Using fruit juices with unflavored gelatin gives you the food value of the juice plus its natural sweet flavor.

1 (12 oz.) can frozen juice concentrate, thawed*
3 envelopes unflavored gelatin
1-1/2 cups (1 can) water

Soften gelatin in juice concentrate. Boil the water, add the juice/gelatin mixture and stir until gelatin dissolves. Remove from heat, pour into a lightly greased square pan and chill. Cut into squares when firm. Refrigerate in a covered container.

*Use orange, apple, grape, cranberry, etc.

CHAPTER 15

The Later Years

YOU WILL LEARN...

1. Various theories on aging and the part nutrition may play.

2. How the cells, organs, and skeleton change in the later years.

3. The special roles of protein, carbohydrate, minerals and vitamins in the older adult's diet.

4. What the effect of caffeine, alcohol, and prescription drugs can be on the body.

5. Practical ways the person alone, no matter at what age, can assure nutritional adequacy with some new ideas and a little bit of planning.

6. What kind of assistance is available for older Americans unable to cope perfectly with every aspect of living.

7. What you can do right now to prepare for a healthy and happy life during your later years.

THE LATER YEARS

1. One out of every _____ persons is about 65 years of age.

2. Older people _____ (are/are not) all poor, lonely, and ill.

3. Two-thirds of the elderly are relatively free of _____ problems.

4. One-third, however, live at or below the _____ line and deserve our attention.

THEORIES ON AGING

5. In the last 25 years there has been _____ (an increase/no increase) in life span. The total life expectancy for any individual is about _____ years.

6. If age is _____, people will claim to be old (Note: venerated means prized, or appreciated)

Aging of Cells

7. Cells seem to age in two ways: by a built-in _____ process, and as a response to outside _____ forces.

8. Aging occurs when the cells become incapable of _____ their constituents.

9. Cells have different timetables for reproduction, but each type of cell seems to come to a _____ end.

10. Thousands of cells die daily in the _____, and there is no mechanism to repair this magnificent instrument.

11. After human cells replicate about 50-55 times, they
     _____.

12. We may also accumulate intracellular "_____" made up
     of partially completed proteins and oxidized lipids that
     are not completely dismantled.

13. The pigment of old age, or aging pigment is called
     _____.

14. If cells lose their ability to interpret the DNA genetic
     code and make incorrect proteins, two things happen:
     a. The body's _____ system will react to them as
         if they are foreign proteins.
     b. Needed proteins will not be supplied where they are
         needed.

15. The autoimmune theory may account in part for the
     accumulation of deposits in joints, which causes
     _____.

16. Cosmic rays may bombard molecules in the cells and split
     them into damaging _____. The
     formation of free radicals might be retarded by the taking
     of vitamin _____ supplements, according to some
     investigators.

Aging of Organs

17. The most visible changes take place in the _____.

18. One reason skin wrinkles is the loss of _____ that
     underlies the skin and also a loss of _____.
     Exposure to sun, wind, and cold hasten the _____
     process.

19. There are changes in other systems including the hair, the
     digestive system, and the _____ and teeth. Also,
     the senses of _____ and _____ diminish.

20. There _____(is/is not) a loss of liver cells but
     _____ gradually reduces the liver's work output by
     infiltrating the cells.

21. All systems are affected by _____ changes in the
     cardiovascular system.

CHAPTER 15:   THE LATER YEARS

22. One thing that promotes maintenance and growth of capillaries is _____.

23. Impaired _____ _____ function causes much unhappiness as it manifests itself in diminished _____ ability, visual _____, hearing _____, and loss of the senses of smell and taste.

24. The quantity of blood pumped by the left ventricle into the aorta each minute is called the _____ _____.

25. The maximum volume of air that can be inhaled into or exhaled from the lungs is called the _____ _____.

Aging of the Skeleton

26. After age _____, bone loss becomes more rapid than bone- _____.

27. Three things that contribute to osteoporosis are:
    1. Low _____ intake or reduced _____ absorption.
    2. _____changes.
    3. Reduced _____ activity.

28. Calcium needs of older women may be as high as _____ mg per day.

NUTRITION IMPLICATIONS OF AGING

29. Good_____ throughout life is the best guarantee of enjoyable later years.

kCalories

30. Energy needs _____ with advancing age.

31. Protein-kcalorie malnutrition is _____ in older people, especially if they have been dieting or eating monotonous diets.

32. Protein foods should contribute about _____ percent of the kcalories in the older person's diet. Fats should contribute no more than _____ percent and the remainder should come from complex _____. All foods should be _____ dense.

33. The rat experiment that severely restricted food early in the animal's life is probably _____ (applicable/not applicable) directly to humans.

Protein

34. Low hemoglobin levels have been shown to correlate with the _____ content of the diet.

35. In one study, only those with excellent _____ had a high protein intake.

Fat

36. _____ should be limited in the older person's diet.

37. High fat intake can interfere with _____ absorption and promote obesity as well as contributing to high levels of _____ in the blood.

Carbohydrate

38. Ways need to be found to increase the consumption of _____ and _____ which are found to be too expensive or too difficult to prepare by some elderly persons.

Vitamins

39. Because so few elderly persons eat the "Basic Four" every day, many _____ and _____ deficiencies are present, greatly contributing to declining health.

40. Some older people use mineral oil or other _____, decreasing _____ absorption.

41. Prescription drugs and antibiotics also interfere with _____ intake or absorption.

42. If the kcalorie intake is below 1,555 per day, it _____ (is/is not) recommended that a vitamin-mineral supplement in the amount of the RDA be taken daily.

Minerals

43. Low blood hemoglobin can result from a diet deficient in _____ (protein/zinc).

44.   Iron deficiency can be worsened by drinking tea, using antacids, blood loss, or reduced stomach _____ secretion.

45.   Another common nutrition problem in older people is a deficiency of _____ which can contribute to the loss of _____ and slowed _____ healing.

46.   Again, _____ deficiency is common and hard to cope with since many persons do not use much milk at all.

47.   Cheese and dried _____ powder, broths made from _____ and other ideas may be useful.

48.   Many medications impair _____ absorption and so does the use of _____.

49.   The use of _____ should be minimized.

50.   Eating "Basic _____" foods every day helps insure _____ sufficiency.

Fiber

51.   Some fibers, with the notable exception of _____ _____, bind cholesterol and carry it out of the body.

52.   Fiber helps prevent the need for _____.

Water

53.   Sufficient _____ is important to help in all bodily functions. Elderly persons tend to be _____ easily as their thirst mechanism is not always reliable.

Caffeine

54.   Caffeine is not _____ but it is habit-_____, and the body adapts to its use to some extent.

55.   An overdose of caffeine produces the same symptoms as an _____ attack.

56.   Very large doses of caffeine have been implicated in causing _____ _____ in people with damaged hearts.

CHAPTER 15: THE LATER YEARS

Alcohol

57. Alcohol has a negative effect on the vitamins _____
     and _____ and on the minerals _____ and
     _____. It may also interfere with nutrient intake.

PRACTICAL POINTERS

Review the ideas of managing mealtimes. They are all applicable
for a busy student on a budget

MEALTIMES ALONE

58. Malnutrition among the elderly is most often due to
     _____.

59. The pressing need seems to be for _____ first,
     then for _____.

60. Apathy evolves from _____. Apathy saps
     energy and nutrient deficiencies develop that increase
     apathy and depression and result in mental
     _____.

61. Vitamin deficiency can be misdiagnosed as
     _____.

MONEY AND OTHER WORRIES

62. Forced to practice economy, the older person usually first
     eliminates "luxury" items such as fresh _____,
     vegetables, and _____.

63. Sometimes older persons practice food _____ and
     _____, spending money needlessly.

64. Other serious problems facing some elderly persons are poor
     _____ health, mental _____, and chronic
     _____.

ASSISTANCE PROGRAMS

65. The Food Stamp program and Supplemental Security
    _____ program are two examples of programs providing
    help to those who qualify.

CHAPTER 15:   THE LATER YEARS

66. The Social _____ Act provides an income for many
     persons who have contributed to it during their working
     years.

67. The Older American Act of _____ contains an amendment
     which provides a nutrition program for the elderly.

68. There are sites where congregate meals are served and also
     provision for those who are unable to leave their homes.
     The program for the homebound is known as "_____ ____
     _____."

69. The independence rated highly by those over 65 might not be
     good for their _____.

70. Other ingenious seniors form a "diner's club" or take turns
     preparing _____.

71. Sometimes a nursing home is a _____ solution to what
     is really a _____ problem.

PREPARING FOR THE LATER YEARS

72. If the goal is to arrive at maturity with as healthy a mind
     and body as it is possible to have, then it means
     cultivating good _____ status and maintaining a
     program of daily _____.

73. It is important not to drift into _____, but to
     maintain many _____.

SUMMING UP

Review text as necessary. You might want to think how this
information could apply to your parents, your grandparents, or
other elderly relatives. It is also important to realize how
your present eating patterns might affect your own later years.

ANSWERS

1. nine
2. are not
3. major
4. poverty
5. no increase, 70
6. venerated
7. genetic, environmental
8. replenishing
9. natural
10. brain
11. die
12. sludge
13. lipofuscin
14. a. immune
15. arthritis
16. free radicals, E
17. skin
18. fat, elasticity, aging
19. bones, taste, smell
20. is not, fat
21. degenerative
22. exercise
23. nerve cell, mental, impairment, loss
24. cardiac index
25. vital capacity
26. 40, building
27. 1. calcium, calcium
    2. hormonal
    3. physical
28. 1,000
29. nutrition
30. decrease
31. common
32. 12-20, 30, carbohydrates, nutrient
33. not applicable
34. protein

35. teeth
36. Fat
37. calcium, cholesterol
38. fruits, vegetables
39. vitamin, mineral
40. laxatives, vitamin
41. vitamin
42. is
43. protein
44. acid
45. zinc, taste, wound
46. calcium
47. milk, bones
48. calcium, alcohol
49. salt
50. Four, nutrient
51. wheat bran
52. laxatives
53. water, dehydrated
54. addictive, forming
55. anxiety
56. heart attacks
57. thiamin, folacin, calcium, zinc
58. loneliness
59. companionship, food
60. loneliness, confusion
61. senility
62. fruits, milk
63. fads, fallacies
64. dental, illness, alcoholism
65. Income
66. Security
67. 1965
68. Meals on Wheels
69. health
70. meals
71. medical, social
72. nutrition, exercise
73. isolation, contacts

SELF TEST

1. If there were 81 persons in attendance at a lecture of public interest, it could be expected that _____ of them would be over age 65 if this sample group followed the national average in the United States.
    a. three
    b. five
    c. seven
    d. nine
    e. eleven

2. Most elderly people live in nursing or convalescent homes.
    a. true
    b. false

3. Because of the failure of our society to provide adequately for the elderly, the majority are poor, lonely and ill.
    a. true
    b. false

4. The percentage of elderly persons living at or below the poverty level is about:
    a. one-third.
    b. one-half.
    c. two thirds.
    d. eighty percent.

5. In the last 25 years there has been _____ in life expectancy for people who are already 20 years of age or older.
    a. a 25% increase
    b. a 10% increase
    c. no increase
    d. a 50% increase

6. The life expectancy for an individual according to statistics is approximately _____ of age.
    a. 60 years
    b. 70 years
    c. 80 years
    d. 90 years
    e. none of the above

7. If an aged person is venerated, the following might be true:
    a. they are prized and honored.
    b. they are ignored.
    c. they disgust or sicken people.
    d. none of the above

8. The aging of cells seems to be:
    a. genetic.
    b. cnvironmental.
    c. to be caused by lack of nutrients.
    d. a and b
    e. b and c

9. Theories of aging include all but:
    a. at some point the cells become incapable of replenishing themselves.
    b. aging cells are programmed to stop reproducing once a certain stage of development has been reached.
    c. cells become cluttered with debris.
    d. cells lose the ability to make the correct proteins.
    e. all of the above statements are correct.

10. The aging of cells is most visible in the:
    a. hair.
    b. skin.
    c. digestive system.
    d. liver.

11. Lipofuscin is known as:
    a. the fusion of two lipids after absorption.
    b. the cardiac sphincter.
    c. the DNA code for lipids.
    d. the growing together of two vertebrae.
    e. the pigment of old age.

12. The adult RDA for calcium is:
    a. 500 mg.
    b. 700 mg.
    c. 800 mg.
    d. 1,000 mg.
    e. none of the above

13. To prevent the development of osteoporosis one needs to:
    a. increase calcium to 1,000 mg. at menopause.
    b. have a lifelong adequate supply of calcium.
    c. have a lifelong adequate intake of fluoride.
    d. schedule physical workouts as part of a regular routine.
    e. all of the above

14. Energy needs _____ with advancing age.
    a. increase
    b. decrease
    c. stay the same

15. The need for essential amino acids lessens considerably during the aging process.
    a. true
    b. false

16. The group of food most neglected by old people is the:
    a. milk group.
    b. meat group.
    c. fruit and vegetable group.
    d. bread and cereal group.

17. Which of the following contributes to iron-deficiency anemia?
    a. Drinking tea.
    b. Using antacids.
    c. A low calorie diet that lacks color.
    d. Reduced stomach acid secretion.
    e. all of the above

18. A large dose of caffeine could cause all the following except:
    a. an anxiety attack.
    b. extra heartbeats.
    c. development of atherosclerosis.
    d. recurring headaches.
    e. heart attacks in people with damaged hearts.

19. Malnutrition among the elderly is most often due to:
    a. loneliness.
    b. lack of education.
    c. poor housing.
    d. multiple disabilities.
    e. retirement.

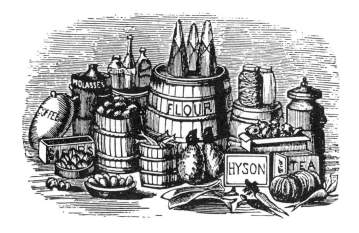

ANSWERS

1. d
2. b
3. b
4. a
5. c
6. b
7. a
8. d
9. e
10. b
11. e
12. c
13. e
14. b
15. b
16. c
17. c
18. c
19. a

HOBO DINNER PACKS

Many people living alone avoid variety in meals because they don't want more dishes to wash. Here are some ideas for solving that problem.

Place one of the following in center of foil square about 12" x 12":

CHICKEN: One piece of chicken. Add 2 tbsp catsup or 2 tbsp orange juice, or 1 tsp soy sauce mixed with 1 tbsp of water and 1 tbsp of honey.

HAMBURGER: 1/4 pound ground chuck mixed with 2 tbsp cracker crumbs, 1/4 tsp onion flakes. Add one of these: 2 tbsp catsup or 2 tbsp water mixed with 1 bouillon cube (to dissolve cube) or 2 tbsp tomato sauce with a pinch of oregano and a pinch of basil or 1 slice of American cheese plus 1 tbsp of milk.

FISH: 1 filet of fish. Add 1 tbsp of butter, 1 tsp of lemon juice.

PLANNED OVERS: One serving of leftover meat or casserole main dish. Fold foil edges in double fold and seal ends.

VEGETABLE HOBO PACK: Place 1/4 package of frozen vegetable in center of foil square. Add seasonings.

FRUIT DUMPLING PACK: Place 1 tbsp butter or margarine and 2 tbsp of brown sugar in center of foil square. Add 1/2 cup of fruit (or 1/2 peach, pear or another fruit). Sprinkle with cinnamon or other spices if desired. Top with 2 refrigerator biscuits.

Seal the packs carefully! Fold the edges together and be sure to seal the ends.

STEAMED CUSTARD PUDDING

1/3 cup powdered milk	1 cup water
2 eggs	3 tbsp sugar
dash of salt	1/2 tsp of vanilla flavoring
nutmeg	

Mix or blend all ingredients either in mixing bowl, or in blender jar. Pour into 2 six-ounce custard cups. Sprinkle nutmeg on top of each custard. Steam (uncovered) with Hobo Packs.

Method of Steaming Hobo Packs

Place all sealed Hobo Packs and custards in large skillet containing 3/4 inch of water. Cover skillet, place on high heat. When water boils reduce heat to simmer. If uncooked foods are in packets, steam for 40-60 minutes (depends upon serving sizes); if pre-cooked foods are being reheated, steam for 25-40 minutes (depends upon whether foods are taken from the refrigerator or freezer).

Try other foods in this method. With experience, your favorite foods can be prepared in this manner without scorching foods and with easy clean-up after the meal.

SOME OTHER SIMPLE IDEAS FOR LUNCH

Omelet with toast and fruit.
Toasted cheese sandwich with grapefruit salad and french
    dressing or tossed salad with mandarin oranges.
Bean soup with chopped fish and celery sandwich.
Cream of pea soup with liverwurst and lettuce sandwich.
Chicken soup with tomato and cucumber sandwich.
Chopped egg sandwich on whole wheat bread, add a coleslaw or
    fresh spinach salad.
Clam chowder, whole wheat crackers, banana and orange slices.
Cream of chicken soup with apple and celery salad.
Scoop of cottage cheese on lettuce with a combination of fresh
    or canned fruit served with hot rolls, muffins or toast.
Deviled eggs, cold leftover sliced meatloaf, chicken or roast,
    served with carrot salad.
Creamed eggs on toast, raw vegetable salad (don't forget to
    add leftover peas, beans, carrots, etc.)

Self Study Forms

FORM 1 Nutrient Intakes (Use One Form for Each Day)

Food	Approximate Measure or Weight	Energy[a] (kcal)	Protein[b] (g)	Fat[b] (g)	Carbo-hydrate[b] (g)	Calcium[a] (mg)	Iron[c] (mg)	Zinc[b] (mg)	Vitamin A[a] (RE)	Thiamin[c] (mg)	Riboflavin[c] (mg)	Niacin[b] (mg)	Folacin[a] (μg)	Vitamin C[b] (mg)
Total														

[a] Compute these values to the nearest whole number.
[b] Compute these values to one decimal place.
[c] Compute these values to two decimal places.

FORM 1   Nutrient Intakes (Use One Form for Each Day)

Food	Approximate Measure or Weight	Energy[a] (kcal)	Protein[b] (g)	Fat[b] (g)	Carbo-hydrate[b] (g)	Calcium[a] (mg)	Iron[c] (mg)	Zinc[b] (mg)	Vitamin A[a] (RE)	Thiamin[c] (mg)	Riboflavin[c] (mg)	Niacin[b] (mg)	Folacin[a] (μg)	Vitamin C[b] (mg)
Total														

[a] Compute these values to the nearest whole number.
[b] Compute these values to one decimal place.
[c] Compute these values to two decimal places.

FORM 1 Nutrient Intakes (Use One Form for Each Day)

Food	Approximate Measure or Weight	Energy[a] (kcal)	Protein[b] (g)	Fat[b] (g)	Carbo-hydrate[b] (g)	Calcium[a] (mg)	Iron[c] (mg)	Zinc[b] (mg)	Vitamin A[a] (RE)	Thiamin[c] (mg)	Riboflavin[c] (mg)	Niacin[b] (mg)	Folacin[a] (μg)	Vitamin C[b] (mg)
Total														

[a] Compute these values to the nearest whole number.
[b] Compute these values to one decimal place.
[c] Compute these values to two decimal places.

FORM 2 Average Daily Energy and Nutrient Intakes

Day	Energy (kcal)	Protein (g)	Fat (g)	Carbo-hydrate (g)	Calcium (mg)	Iron (mg)	Zinc (mg)	Vitamin A (RE)	Thiamin (mg)	Riboflavin (mg)	Niacin (mg)	Folacin (µg)	Vitamin C (mg)
1													
2													
3													
Total													
Average daily intake (divide total by 3)													

FORM 3 Comparison with a Standard Intake

Day	Energy (kcal)	Protein (g)	Fat (g)	Carbo-hydrate (g)	Calcium (mg)	Iron (mg)	Zinc (mg)	Vitamin A (RE)	Thiamin (mg)	Riboflavin (mg)	Niacin (mg)	Folacin (µg)	Vitamin C (mg)
Average daily intake (from Form 2)													
Standard[a]													
Intake as percentage of standard[b]													

[a] Taken from RDA tables (inside front cover) or *Recommended Nutrient Intakes for Canadians* (Appendix O).
[b] For example, if your intake of protein was 50 g and the standard for a person your age and sex was 46 g, then you consumed $(50 \div 46) \times 100$, or 109 percent of the standard.

FORM 4 Percentage of kCalories from Protein, Fat, and Carbohydrate

From Form 3:
Protein: _____ g/day × 4 kcal/g = (P)_____ kcal/day
Fat: _____ g/day × 9 kcal/g = (F)_____ kcal/day
Carbohydrate: _____ g/day × 4 kcal/g = (C)_____ kcal/day
Total kcal/day = (T)_____ kcal/day

Percentage of kcalories from protein:
$$\frac{(P)}{(T)} \times 100 = \text{\_\_\_\_\_ \% of total kcalories}$$

Percentage of kcalories from fat:
$$\frac{(F)}{(T)} \times 100 = \text{\_\_\_\_\_ \% of total kcalories}$$

Percentage of kcalories from carbohydrate:
$$\frac{(C)}{(T)} \times 100 = \text{\_\_\_\_\_ \% of total kcalories}$$

Note: The three percentages can total 99, 100, or 101, depending on the way in which figures were rounded off earlier.

FOOD GROUP AND RECOMMENDED INTAKE	YOUR INTAKE FROM GROUP (SPECIFY FOOD AND AMOUNT)	YOUR SCORE
Fruits and vegetables—4 or more portions (½ cup cooked edible portion or 3–4 oz, 100 g, raw); at least 1 raw daily		
1 portion vitamin A–rich dark green or deep orange fruit or vegetable (any food with more than your RDA) = 10 points (no more than 10 points allowed)		
1 portion vitamin C–rich fruit or vegetable (any food with more than your RDA) = 10 points (no more than 10 points allowed)		
Other fruits and vegetables, incuding potatoes = 2.5 each		
Subtotal (no more than 25 points allowed)		
Breads and cereals—4 or more portions of whole-grain or enriched (1 oz dry-weight cereal or 1-oz slice bread or equivalent grain product)		
1 portion cereal or 2 bread equivalents = 10 points (no more than 10 points allowed)		
Other bread equivalents = 5 points each		
Subtotal (no more than 25 points allowed)		
Milk and milk products—2 or more portions (8 oz fluid milk; calcium equivalents are 1⅓ oz hard cheese, 1⅓ c cottage cheese, 1 pint ice milk or ice cream)		
One portion = 12.5 points		
Subtotal (no more than 25 points allowed)		
Meat and meat substitutes—2 or more portions of meat (2–3 oz of cooked lean meat, fish, poultry; protein equivalents are 2 eggs, 2 oz hard cheese, or ½ c cottage cheese) and 2 portions legumes or nuts (¾ c cooked legumes, 4 tbsp peanut butter, 1 oz nuts or sunflower seeds); count cheese either in milk group or in meat group, not both		
2 portions meat = 12.5 points		
2 portions legumes = 12.5 points		
Subtotal (no more than 25 points allowed)		
Grand total (no more than 100 points)		

The above are foundation foods. Additional foods are those that do not fit into the above groupings but add flavor, interest, variety, and (often) kcalories. List those eaten:

_____   _____   _____
_____   _____   _____
_____   _____   _____

FORM 6 Minutes Spent at Each Energy Level

CLOCK TIME	TOTAL MINUTES	ACTIVITY	a	b	c	d	e	f
					ENERGY LEVEL[a]			
7:00 – 7:45	45	Dressing		8	23	14		
7:45 – 8:15	30	Eating		26	4			
8:15 – 9:00	45	Biking to school			4	25	16	

(Stairs: up _I_
           down _II_   )

Total

[a] See Table 6–2 for an explanation of these levels.

387

FORM 7   Energy Cost for Muscular Activities (Exclusive of Basal Metabolism and the Effect of Food)

ENERGY LEVEL	TOTAL MINUTES SPENT		ENERGY COST PER MINUTE (KCAL/KG/MIN)			TOTAL ENERGY COST PER KG (KCAL/KG)
			Women	Men		
a		×	0.000	0.000	=	0.000
b		×	0.001–0.007	0.003–0.012	=	
c		×	0.009–0.016	0.014–0.022	=	
d		×	0.018–0.035	0.023–0.040	=	
e		×	0.036–0.053	0.042–0.060	=	
f		×	0.055	0.062		
Subtotal	1,440					
Extra energy spent on stairs:						
Flights down		×	0.012		=	
Flights up		×	0.036		=	
Total kcal/kg/24 hours						

Now multiply by body weight (kg) to arrive at total energy spent on activities for the day:	×	kg
	=	kcal/day

FOOD I ATE	PORTION OR AMOUNT	EXCHANGE LIST	NUMBER OF EXCHANGES
Banana	1 medium	fruit	2

FORM 9 kCalories Consumed in One Day Based on Exchanges

EXCHANGE LIST	TOTAL EXCHANGES	× KCAL/EXCHANGE =	ENERGY (KCAL)
Milk[a]		× 80 =	
Vegetables		× 25 =	
Fruit		× 40 =	
Bread		× 70 =	
Meat[b]		× 55 =	
Fat		× 45 =	
Sugar, tsp.		× 20 =	
		Total:	kcal

[a] If you used whole milk, add 2 fats for each cup of milk you drank. If you used low-fat milk, add 1 fat for each cup.
[b] If you used high-fat meat, add 1 fat for each ounce of meat. If you used medium-fat meat, add ½ fat for each ounce.

FORM 10 Diet Planning by Exchange Groups TH7-2

		Amounts to be Delivered[b]			
Exchange List	Number of Exchanges[a]	Carbohydrate ——— g	Protein ——— g	Fat ——— g	Energy[c] ——— kcal
Milk					
Vegetable					
Fruit					
Bread					
Meat					
Fat					
	Total actually delivered				

[a] From steps 4, 5, 6.
[b] From step 3.
[c] From step 7.

FORM 11 Meal Patterns TH7-3

EXCHANGE LIST	TOTAL EXCHANGES TO BE CONSUMED DAILY[a]	EXCHANGES CONSUMED AT EACH MEAL				
		BREAKFAST	LUNCH	SNACK	DINNER	SNACK
Milk						
Vegetable						
Fruit						
Bread						
Meat						
Fat						

[a] From Form 7-1, column 2.

FORM 12 Nutrient Density of a Food

Food chosen for analysis _____

	Energy (kcal)	Protein (g)	Calcium (mg)	Iron (mg)	Zinc (mg)	Vitamin A (RE)	Thiamin (mg)	Riboflavin[a] (mg)	Folacin (µg)	Vitamin C (mg)
① Your recommended intake										
② Amount provided by one serving of the food										
Percentage of recommended intake provided by one serving	③ Comparison number	④								④
⑤ Nutrition score										

⑥ Is the food nutritious? _____

[a] A complete calculation would include niacin, but we have omitted it because of the difficulty in estimating niacin derived from tryptophan (see Chapter 8).

FORM 13 Calculating the Relative Costs of Protein

	REGULAR HAMBURGER	LOW-FAT MILK	PLAIN CORNFLAKES	PEANUT BUTTER	EGGS	CANNED PORK AND BEANS
Grams protein per measure	23 g / 3 oz			4 g / 1 tbsp		
Amount of food to provide 10 g protein						
Cost of unit amount of food						
Cost of amount of food to provide 10 g protein						
Cost of 1 g protein						

†